YOU CAN
FIX THE FAT
FROM CHILDHOOD
& Other Heart Disease Risks, Too

Gerald S. Berenson, MD
NancyKay Sullivan Wessman, MPH

authorHOUSE®

AuthorHouse™
1663 Liberty Drive
Bloomington, IN 47403
www.authorhouse.com
Phone: 1-800-839-8640

Published by AuthorHouse 8/29/2012

ISBN: 978-1-4772-5783-8 (e)
ISBN: 978-1-4772-5784-5 (hc)
ISBN: 978-1-4772-5785-2 (sc)

Library of Congress Control Number: 2012914755

This book recognizes all the dedicated researchers,
nurses and staff, educational professionals,
parents, and children
in Bogalusa and Franklinton, Louisiana,
who have participated in the Bogalusa Heart Study
and the Health Ahead/Heart Smart Program

Contents

Illustrations

*Used with permission of Tulane University, Donn Young,
photographer*

Bogalusa Heart Study
*Used with permission, PBurch/Tulane University
Publications*

"The weight of the nation is out of control, but we can fix that."

Shiriki K. Kumanyika, PhD, MPH
Associate Dean, Professor
University of Pennsylvania School of Medicine

As Seen on HBO "The Weight Of The Nation"

Preface

Why write a book like this? Obesity has come along and forced almost everyone to think about its dangers. Above-average fatness has stimulated – no, *urged* – us to see what we can do to help prevent obesity in young children who are rapidly becoming obese. We want to help you and your family achieve healthier lifestyles, lose weight if needed, and prevent the risk of heart disease and diabetes.

Many books exist – look at the number of cookbooks and books on health. What gives us the right, the credibility, to try to develop our messages to help you and your family and children lead a healthier life? We are not trying to push anti-obesity drugs or bariatric surgery or special diets, although these are, in some instances, appropriate.

But we have been at it a long time – we being Berenson, the founder, and many other individuals who have worked over the years and contributed to the Bogalusa Heart Study. We have seen and treated the medical problems; we have learned how all this begins in childhood; we have done a lot of research; and we think we know some preventive measures that work – and we are open to change. We want to help.

If you are a parent, teacher, community leader, or individual concerned about improved health for your family, this book will help you. **You Can Fix The Fat From Childhood — & Other Heart Disease Risks, Too** promotes family-focused comprehensive heart health knowledge and behaviors so that you and your family can achieve the best health. You can improve how you feel and think about yourself. You can adjust whether you yourself or someone else in your family becomes or remains fat, and you can prevent heart disease. You can learn to work with health and education professionals toward reducing disability from heart disease and, maybe, prolong life and quality of life.

Observations over the many years in the Bogalusa Heart Study have established that adverse cardiovascular risk factors begin early in life. Multiple long term pediatric studies have clearly established that adult heart diseases begin in childhood. Through findings from the most detailed and long term studies – the Muscatine Study, Finnish Youth Study, and the Bogalusa Heart Study – we know that prevention of adult cardiovascular disease must begin early. We call it primordial prevention, *before* bad risk factors begin and result in heart disease and related diseases, like diabetes.

So, read and think about what we have written. Learn healthier lifestyles, healthy decision-making, "choices," and bring your kids along.

One of the first steps to take toward preventing too early disease and death is to decide to tackle the fat. Prevent it, control it, exercise it. When one, a thousand, 10 million individuals take(s) action to become healthier, the population becomes healthier. You have taken the first step.

Introduction

Am I fat? Does this outfit make me look big? Why do they call me Fatso? When and how did this happen to me? Am I and my family following healthy lifestyles? Are my children growing up fit, physically and mentally?

You – facing the facts of fat, knowing you did it to yourself and feeling frustrated. Whether you are female or male, 20-something or in your 40s, dark- or light-skinned, most people crave to be slim, trim, toned, and fit.

You and your family can be, but we are not all born with the body of a performance athlete. Health doesn't come in a bottle, and you cannot buy it in a drug store or at the supermarket! You have to work at it. You and your kids can earn it.

This book focuses on fatness as one of the most important risk factors for heart disease. This comes from 40 years of studying children as they've aged, grown fatter over time, and developed risk factors leading to such chronic conditions as hypertension, high blood cholesterol, and diabetes. Along with smoking and physical inactivity, those "risk factors" lead to chronic diseases that kill or disable seven of every 10 people in the United States, adversely affecting the quality of life of some 90 million Americans. Risk factors and poor lifestyles that cause these ills begin in childhood.

Research scientists involved in the Bogalusa Heart Study proved that risk factors are detectable in early childhood. We have documented physical heart and vascular changes by the time children reach five to eight years of age. We have shown how children can be measured in the same way as adults or for people who are already too sick to achieve a maximum benefit from prevention. We refer to you, but that includes your family. You can provide the leadership to a healthier life.

If you live in the United States or another industrialized country of the West, chances are two-to-one that you are overweight. Same holds true for teens and youngsters, too. Two-thirds of the people who live in the U.S. are overweight or obese, according to the Centers for Disease Control and Prevention. Ten percent of children from two through five years of age, nearly 20 percent of those six to 11, and almost as many from 12 to 19 years also are medically classified as obese.

Chances are, in relation to your health future, "The horses are already out of the barn." The old saying indicates you've already grown beyond the ideal weight for men or women your age; check the charts for your children in this book. Though you might never knowingly participate in risky behavior – never taking part in extreme sports or unprotected sex, for example – you might already be among the 67 percent of Americans who are overweight or obese. You represent *risky* business.

Being fat or morbidly obese with no thought toward change guarantees health problems, especially heart disease. Being fat, especially in childhood, ranks as one of the top six risk factors for heart disease.

But you can reduce the risk factors for yourself and, over time and with determination, help your family become heart-healthy.

Most people who have developed heart disease risk factors can benefit by healthy lifestyle and treatment, but think how much better every individual's health would be if prevention started in childhood, if everyone developed and exhibited a mindset for the body to be healthy. Simply, prevention is learning how to follow healthy lifestyles! Learn about primordial prevention.

You Can Fix The Fat From Childhood — & Other Heart Disease Risks, Too concisely pulls together information that can guide your family to discover risk factors and understand how you can avoid or reduce the effects of those risks through childhood, adolescence, young adulthood, middle age, and the late years of life. Adults can learn to change the health of children and teens positively before disease becomes an issue. Importantly, children can learn to achieve a healthy existence for life!

The observations are based on scientific evidence gathered over time. The lessons certainly apply generally. It's like putting money into a bank or investing for interest for future use. Genetics and family heredity obviously play a big part and cannot be changed, but we as individuals and families can control environmental impact, lifestyles, and our behavior. Sure, genetics is important. You are born with it and cannot change it, but read about the importance of environment, culture, and lifestyles.

Why write a book like this? We have been at it for over four decades. We practice clinical medicine and see the ravages of heart disease. We know the cost. We see and have endured the emotional trauma. We have done the research and are beginning to understand prevention. We can't cure heart disease or prevent death – that is the natural course of living. But we can delay that eventuality and perhaps improve quality of life. We are dedicated based on studies to help.

Perhaps we include too many facts, but these are the basis of our recommendations. Excuse us for having restatements or overlap in messages or ideas. We might be too disinclined to correct, but my head of medicine professor used to say in teaching us to teach medical students, "If you keep slinging mud at the barn door, some of it will stick."

Individuals can live healthfully with fun, a better attitude, more energy, and improved fitness. Best to start at birth, although even adults can lose weight, exercise, practice healthy behaviors, and achieve better health. Reclaiming optimum health – losing extra pounds to achieve "normal" weight – requires a complex recipe of attitude and actions. Losing weight can feel like hard work and involves change; it's not fast or easy, but you can do it.

Chapter One
The Bogalusa Heart Study

In 1972, the Bogalusa Heart Study (BHS, Bogalusa, Louisiana) was identified at Louisiana State University (LSU) Medical Center as a national Specialized Center of Research (SCOR). The United States Congress had mandated the National Institutes of Health to establish SCORs to investigate major causes of cardiovascular disease: atherosclerosis — a generic term for heart and vascular changes, hypertension, pulmonary disease, strokes, and thrombosis.

Bogalusa Heart Study is the only long-term, cardiovascular, community research program in the world in which both African-American and Caucasian individuals have consistently participated from early childhood through adulthood and middle life. The Study encompassed clinical, epidemiologic, and experimental programs on atherosclerosis, essential hypertension, and diabetes as they related to later coronary and hypertensive heart diseases – and also how these begin in childhood. Before, no comprehensive examination of all children in a total biracial (black and white) community had been undertaken with this detail.

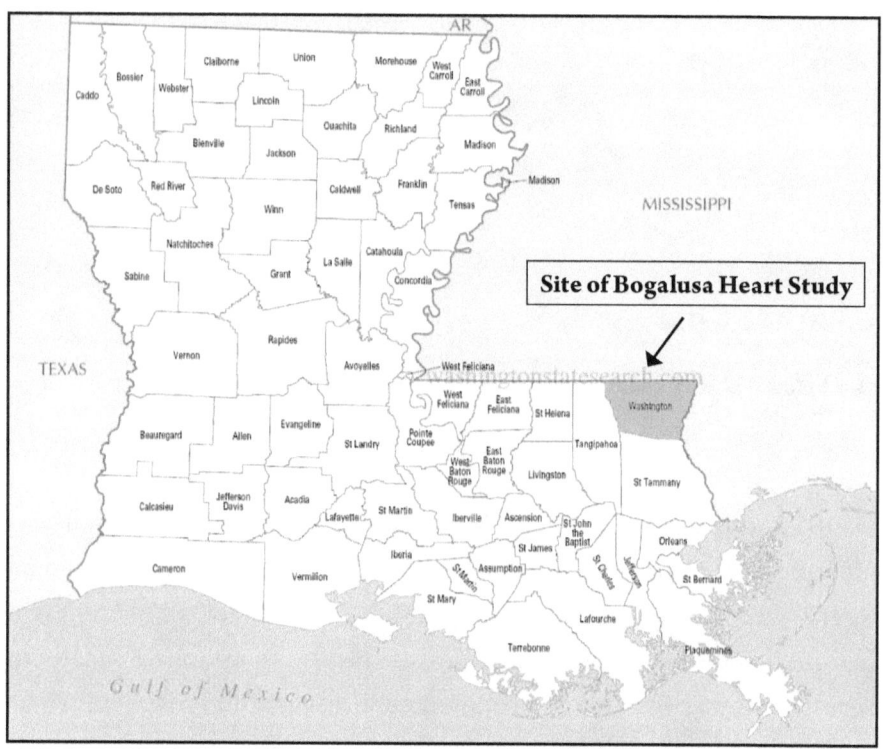

Louisiana and Washington Parish

The Study – which began at LSU School of Medicine in 1972 and moved to become the flagship Tulane University Center for Cardiovascular Health, Disease, and Prevention in 1991 – brought together a highly skilled and trained, multi-disciplinary team of anthropologists, biochemists, cardiologists, epidemiologists, geneticists, nurses, nutritionists, psychologists, sociologists, statisticians, and – *finally* – school teachers. They worked together to study hereditary and environmental aspects of early coronary artery disease (CAD), hypertension, and diabetes. Funding for the research came from the National Heart, Lung, and Blood Institute, the National Institute for Child Health and Human Development, the National Institute of Aging, and the American Heart Association – *basically* from taxpayers like you and volunteers.

The Bogalusa Heart Study focus was to understand the early natural history of coronary artery disease (atherosclerosis or hardening of the arteries), essential hypertension (high blood pressure), and diabetes mellitus (abnormally high glucose levels in the blood). Our researchers aimed to address these questions in designing and beginning the Study of children five to 17 years. As time allowed in the research, the ages were extended to both and recently to 45 years of age to look at aging and longevity. More information is available at www.tulane.edu/som/cardiohealth.

Researchers had four fundamental questions that guided the beginning of the BHS.

- What is the distribution and prevalence of cardiovascular risk factors in children? How are risk factors defined in childhood? What levels of risk factor variables in children are abnormal? We now know a lot about the normal and abnormal levels, how they are measured, and how they produce a life-long burden on the cardiovascular system, importantly beginning in childhood.

- What are the interrelationships of risk factors during childhood? Are the relationships similar to those in adults – for example, does obesity relate to hypertension? How do the risk factor observations relate to a child's family history? We now know the risk factors interrelate; obesity is the main culprit, and a family history is very important, as are lifestyles and health behaviors. As you will see, this interrelation is the basis of the metabolic syndrome – the apple, poor body configuration.

- What are the time-course changes of risk factors in children? What are trends during children's growth phases? Are the risk factor levels during childhood predictive of future levels? First of all, risk factors in children do predict those in adulthood; they "track" – high and low levels tend to persist, and they change with growth periods of early childhood, at puberty and adolescence, and in adulthood. Thus, we look at percentiles at different ages and for boys and girls – like the 5th percentile or 95th percentile, which can be abnormal. "Cut points," specific or selected high or low levels from adult heart disease studies, don't apply to growing children. Now we are looking at aging and longevity, and some of our children (500) have died.

- What determines risk factors in children? Simply, why do some children have high levels of risk factors while others have low levels? What is the extent of genetic and environmental determinants? We suffer through or are gratified by having a good genetic (familial) background, but we all have to relate to our environment and respond by lifestyles we choose.

The basis of our Study is genetics versus environment – *read on.*

The BHS took a look at increasing obesity and "superobesity" (morbid obesity) among youngsters in the early 1980s – two decades *before* most people observed the bulge. Even then, America's children were growing fatter, not fitter.

Now CDC calls the problem "common, serious, and costly," about $150 million a year by 2010. That's a hefty price to pay – a huge part of the country's public health and medical dollars going to a human difficulty that can be both predicted and prevented.

We know – we have observed and we have proved in the BHS – that obesity and other major causes of adult heart disease begin in childhood. And we know from a Dutch philosopher's proclamation some 500 years ago and restated by Benjamin Franklin in the 18th century that prevention costs less than cure.

Think back to your own child's earliest days – or infants in general.

Do you remember your child's birth – how absolutely amazed you were to hold such a tiny creature, complete with 10 fingers and 10 toes? Suddenly, the rest of the world simply stopped. That special moment included only you and your baby.

Time could not freeze that moment, however; so you and your child began a journey of teaching and learning from each other. Your child was as risk-free then as he or she would ever be – and we can help children stay that way if we start heart-healthy training from the cradle.

Most newborn babies come into the world healthy.

More than four million infants are born each year, and only a very small percentage suffers heart defects or other diseases. Even so, a staggering 90 percent will develop some aspect of heart and vascular disease.

Using research findings and the closely related comprehensive health promotion program called "Health Ahead/Heart Smart," this book focuses on helping families avoid heart disease. You and individual family members can *choose* to take responsibility for your own good health and for the health of your children.

Books and other material resources about health and growing up to live healthy abound. Many physicians, scientists, public health experts, pop-culture authors, and would-be authorities write books and articles on nutrition and dietary recommendations. The Internet continues to offer ever more options on how individuals can avoid unhealthy risk factors. Advertisers tempt with quick fixes, often including special diets, nutrition plans, and "the magic bullet." Many people believe that information is accurate and will work. But that is not always the case.

If risk factors are uncontrollable, then the doctors need to address the problem. We now have marvelous drugs, and we are learning how to use them for children, if needed. The focus should be not only on adults but also on pre-school, kindergarten, and school-age children.

Observations made over the past 40 years in the BHS clearly show that children manifest "silent" evidence of adult heart disease. Believe it; it's real. Kids with hypertensive heart disease is common – not just a special occurrence but part of early life, maybe 5 to 10 percent. High serum total cholesterol, high blood pressure, obesity, and tobacco use occur in the early years of life and are predictive of future adult illnesses. By the year 2030, unless drastic lifestyle changes occur in homes across the country, heart disease will claim 1.5 million of today's children in the U.S. each year.

The idea that cardiovascular risk factors are detectable in childhood and, therefore, predictive of future risk clearly sets the stage for developing prevention programs at young ages. Yes, *prevention* programs.

Serious risk factors include high cholesterol, the various lipoprotein cholesterols (the good and the bad), high blood pressure, obesity, and aberrations of sugar and insulin metabolism.

Arteriosclerosis includes atherosclerosis (coronary, cerebral, and other vessels in the body) and the cardiovascular system changes related to high blood pressure, with diabetes accelerating both. Diabetes involves changes on very small blood vessels, even in the eyes and kidneys. All these diseases have different and some overlapping changes in the heart and blood vessels, which keep scientists busy and trying to understand how they occur. We are learning more all the time; your concern is to achieve a lifestyle that will prevent or delay them from occurring and also to help your children to grow up healthy.

Atherosclerosis refers to the cholesterol, good and bad lipoproteins, clotting, and causing fibrous changes to occur in blood vessels – coronary vessels that supply the heart, the kidney, the brain, and special vessels or arteries all over the body. Hypertension is the pressure inside blood vessels – not *hyper*-tension, excitement, or anxiety under usual day-to-day conditions but rather tension or blood vessel physical stress that occurs with each heartbeat. Diabetes is an imbalance of sugar being metabolized by cells and how insulin and other hormones work.

And all this begins in childhood, especially with obesity and a family history of diabetes. This is serious, demanding attention and action now.

Chapter Two
Heart disease starts in childhood – *really!*

After 40 years of heart-related research focused on the people in one small community, the question often comes: "What have you learned?" *This is it!*

Almost everyone has heard a variation on the story of a man who goes for a physical examination, passes with flying colors, and then dies of a heart attack on his way home.

And women? Heart diseases claim women, too – more than 35 percent of American women's deaths link to cardiovascular disease. At older ages, women suffer more heart attacks than men, in part because more men have died off.

Every year, 450,000 seemingly healthy Americans die suddenly from massive heart attacks that strike with no warning. In 2004, some 654,000 U.S. citizens – 222.7 per 100,000 people – died of heart disease. Many of the victims never had any inkling that their arteries were clogged and their hearts in mortal danger. Some 50 percent are classified as "sudden death" victims because they do not get to the hospital before dying. Fortunately, emergency programs, CPR training, and emergency defibrillators even at airports and in classrooms are becoming available to address this problem.

Some people worry needlessly about heart trouble when the real cause of their chest pain might be nothing more than indigestion or a pulled muscle. Chest pain might also signal another condition – gall bladder disease or pleurisy, with inflammation of the lining of the lung that can follow a viral infection.

Absent a set of definitive guidelines for diagnosing heart disease, few if any can predict precisely when, how, and why heart attacks occur. No single "thing" causes heart disease. No bacteria, no virus can be directly charged as responsible for atherosclerosis or hypertension. Heart attacks remain non-contagious. But they happen so often, *heart disease is epidemic* — and the subtle process begins in childhood. Heart disease has replaced infectious diseases as the whole world's number one killer.

Additionally, research shows that many victims of heart disease experience low blood flow to the heart – called ischemia – and might feel no pain.

While one episode of ischemia can cause little or no damage to the heart muscle, repeated episodes can lead to fatal heart attacks. Ischemia can occur at any time – when an individual is reading, talking, or even just sitting on the front porch petting the dog. The chest pain called angina pectoris, which might equate with heart disease, appears to be a relatively late sign of coronary artery disease. Classically, it does occur with physical activity, a heavy meal, or anxiety and disappears with rest. We BHS researchers learned that autopsies of young individuals dying from traumatic events – mostly, automobile crashes – already show the atherosclerotic disease in coronary vessels, but chest pain does not occur until after significant blockage of the coronary vessel has happened or from blood clotting in the vessel initiated by an atherosclerotic lesion.

Individuals should not begin to worry that their hearts are having a heart attack in silence. One should pay more attention to health and have a profile by professionals.

Bad choices cost too much

A popular news magazine, reporting results of yet another university study, announced that the top killer in America is individuals making dumb decisions to "engage in self-destructive behavior." Such decisions as drinking and driving can result in vehicular deaths; refusing to curb spending and sinking into ever deeper debt can lead to stress, strokes, and lifelong disability; over-eating, not exercising, and consuming non-nutritious food can lead to obesity, diabetes, and heart disease.

Such huge numbers of people related to chronic disease strain the brain's comprehension of the cost. Health organizations estimated in 2008 that the cost of cardiovascular diseases and stroke in the United States was near to $448.5 billion; diabetes alone costs the nation $218 billion a year. Beyond, consider the cost for emotional pain to families.

Those numbers fail to consider the human costs: the pain and suffering from the disease itself plus the social stigmatization and depression often associated with poor health, particularly obesity and cardiovascular disease. *What a challenge!*

Positive choices pay big rewards

Researchers believed that by studying an entire free-living young population, before disease becomes obvious, we could learn how to influence the early natural course of various forms of heart disease. Our findings show the early natural histories of essential hypertension and coronary artery disease vary with both race and gender, and those variations account for some of the differences observed in clinical heart disease in adults.

Hypertension, for example, occurs much more frequently and more severely in black people, yet white males experience more coronary heart disease events (heart attacks) at an earlier age. Black people tend to have more diabetes, and black females experience more severe obesity and more diabetes, beginning even before adolescence.

While social and cultural differences play a role, clues about black people's having more hypertension and white men's having more coronary artery disease obviously relate to underlying genetic susceptibility influenced by environmental factors. Diet and physical activity or cigarette smoking, to which individuals are exposed over time, interact with an individual's intrinsic makeup.

The environmental factors affect clinical risk factors in adults, but do they influence the development of risk factors from childhood? Can we diagnose coronary atherosclerotic lesions in childhood? Can we diagnose hypertension in childhood — can we diagnose hypertensive disease of target organs affected by high blood pressure, such as an enlarged heart, changes in kidney or blood vessels?

Yes – yes to all those questions.

We also know diet and socioeconomic factors are important and need to be considered. Social diversity also plays a part. Attitudes toward health and lifestyles of healthy or unhealthy behaviors affect risk, so encourage your family to develop good attitudes early!

The concept that cardiovascular risk factors can be detected in childhood and, therefore, might predict future risk clearly sets the stage for developing prevention programs at young ages. Although medical and clinical consequences appear only later in life, the mechanisms that lead to atherosclerosis, hypertension, diabetes, and the metabolic syndrome of insulin resistance become obvious in childhood. Don't give up; we will explain some of the terms, and we provide a glossary.

Scientists still do not know the precise initiating factors, but because physicians can identify the earliest determining factors that establish the characteristics of the disease, young people can come closer to actually delaying or preventing heart disease.

The following are critically important:

Lessons Learned From The Bogalusa Heart Study

— Numbers below represent findings as of 2010 —

Obesity
- Children on average are over 12 pounds heavier, though no taller, since 1973, and are continuing to gain weight, over expected, with growth.
- Over 40 percent of children are overweight or obese, many dangerously fat. Some think the solution is bariatric surgery; that depends on the severity of the obesity.
- Obesity in children predicts cardiac enlargement, insulin resistance, and diabetes in adulthood. The appearance of diabetes has increased, even in adolescence.
- Children, on the average, watch TV two to four hours every day; computers and games add to physical inactivity.

Asthma
- Incidence of asthma has increased from seven to 14 percent.
- Asthma and bronchitis persist into adulthood.

Hypertension
- High blood pressure levels in childhood predict hypertension in adulthood.
- Increased left ventricular mass (heart enlargement) is found in children at 90th percentile of blood pressure levels in the general population of children (the top 10 percent).

Lipids, Lipoproteins
- HDL-C decreases dramatically at puberty in white males and stays low; that's the good cholesterol becoming lower.
- LDL-C rises in adolescence and in young adult white males. That is, the lipoprotein cholesterols become more abnormal as children become adults.

Risk Factors

- Gender and racial contrasts occur. African Americans, especially men, suffer more than whites do from severe hypertension and rampant kidney disease.
- Risk factors "cluster" as a cardiometabolic syndrome, the apple - pear body configuration and "deadly quartet" of risk factors.
- Tracking – risk factor levels continue within a high or low rank as children grow and can predict adult levels. As an example, we can add 40 mg/dl of a child's cholesterol level to predict his or her adult level.
- Risk factors also lead to more diabetes in African Americans and coronary artery disease at an earlier age in white males.

Tobacco and Alcohol Use

- Over 30 percent of high school adolescents are regular smokers, more in white girls and persistent alcohol users (below legal age to purchase). These habits are documented to begin in the 3rd grade (age eight years – second graders could not read the questionnaire!) Children do tend to be experimenters!

Diet

- 60 percent exceed dietary cholesterol intake, as recommended by the American Heart Association.
- 80 percent exceed recommended saturated fat intake.
- Excess sodium (Na+) and inadequate potassium (K+) intake increase cardiovascular risk. Our culture has grossly excess sodium exposure.
- Soft drinks and other "empty" calorie sugary snacks contribute to obesity.

Morbidity and Mortality

- 54.7 percent of known information on deaths at a young adult age are unnatural – automobile accidents, violence, and suicide, for example.
- Average age of heart attacks is 51 years in the Bogalusa community.

- Anatomic changes noted by autopsies of children and young adults relate strongly to risk factors – beginning in childhood. The most critical observation in the BHS is that atherosclerosis is seen in coronary arteries – effects of high blood pressure and changes in kidneys are examples – at childhood and in adolescence.
- Abnormal structure and function changes of the cardiovascular system relate to risk factors – already noted in childhood, a prelude to cardiac events as adults.

Social

- 17 percent of pregnancies occur in teenagers who are unwed.
- In many schools, 35 to 46 percent are dropouts and do not finish high school.
- Healthy lifestyles can reverse many poor outcomes.
- Some risk factors in age/family cannot be changed, but most risk factors can.

Tracking predicts changes

Do risk factors track? That is, do risk factors identified in childhood tend to remain at a high or a low level over time? The answer is *"YES!"* The concept of tracking is important since it allows prediction of levels from childhood to adulthood. We use the word "percentile" to rank levels related to a "normal" population to get an idea what might be normal.

The BHS shows that heart disease begins at young ages. Studying human body measurements – such as height, weight, or blood pressure – over time showed that risk factors "track," are consistent, and predict adult disease. For example, an obese child has a high probability of being an obese adult and will likely increase in fatness. The individual's level ranked as a high percentile, and that person will continue to have a high level – or the reverse. Tracking is not perfect but is good enough to consider adult levels, and the amount of tracking varies for different risk factors – high for LDL-C and lower for blood pressure.

From the early 1970s, we followed children with high blood pressure, obesity, and high cholesterol to determine how risk factors changed with age. Examination of children five, eight, and 12 years apart revealed that height, weight, obesity, and cholesterol do change with age and growth of children, as might be expected. But tracking allows predicting future risk at abnormal levels.

Identifying a child at high risk of serious illness, especially one with a family history of such disease, becomes the first step toward prevention.

We examined risk factors regarding heart disease. Autopsies on children who have, sadly, died demonstrated that atherosclerotic fatty streaks are common in blood vessels of children as young as three. As a person ages, more advanced lesions, fibrous plaques, can develop from these fatty streaks. These can progress with blood clot formation. At an older age, clots can lead to a heart attack. Blocked coronary arteries can result in a myocardial infarction (heart attack) or even sudden death.

Not surprisingly, children with unfavorable and potentially harmful risk factors tend to come from families with an increased incidence of heart disease. But increasingly, children without a family history of heart disease can be at risk for hypertension, high cholesterol, obesity, and diabetes.

Between 1973 and 1994, researchers analyzed 4,000 five- to 17-year-olds in each of seven cross-sectional studies; over the years, many were reexamined as they aged. We found disturbing insight: about 11 percent of examined schoolchildren were considered overweight! Overweight schoolchildren were 2.4 times as likely as thinner children to have an elevated level of total cholesterol. Now that level has increased from 11 in the 1980s to 40 percent's being overweight and obese.

Diabetes? No, thank you. Diabetes is a very serious disease. And it, too, begins in childhood. Adult onset, type 2 diabetes, is occurring earlier at childhood ages primarily because of the epidemic of obesity. Soon we will have an epidemic of diabetes due to obesity.

Of the 813 overweight schoolchildren screened, 475 (58 percent) were found to have at least one risk factor for adult illness. If they have one, they are likely to have two or three.

Researchers conclude: Successful prevention and treatment of risk factors in childhood can reduce the incidence of heart disease and other illnesses in adulthood.

You Can Fix The Fat From Childhood — & Other Heart Disease Risks, Too promotes family-focused comprehensive knowledge and behaviors with an eye toward preventing early disability and death from heart disease. Learning to adopt healthy lifestyles – that's prevention!

As a corollary to the Bogalusa Heart Study, we developed effective prevention programs from the findings based on lifestyles and behavior. Application of health education for children in the general public can help abort or at least delay the cardiovascular maladies so common in our society and worldwide. We now emphasize *primordial* prevention – more about that to come. Our hope is that the potential from prevention beginning in childhood will become recognized as an acceptable and common practice. This is our way to address quality of life from its origin and, maybe, extend quality to the end of life.

Chapter Three
What we know about risk factors

Do you know your numbers? You probably know many different telephone numbers, your driver's license and Social Security numbers, your mortgage payment, statistics for sports of interest, birthdays, but do you know the numbers of your own risk factors? If you do not, get a new doctor. Don't just say, "They're normal." All the reports and guidelines recommending levels of risk factors, some from committee members who have not collected data as we have, and guidelines and recommendations are always changing. Earlier, "normal" blood pressure was below 160/90; now we look for 120/70 in adults.

Of all research developments into the cause, treatment, and prevention of heart disease, the most important is the clear demonstration that different cultural patterns, lifestyles, and personal characteristics bring different degrees of risk for eventual heart attack or stroke.

Major risk factors identified to date are obesity in childhood, high blood pressure, high blood cholesterol and other lipids or lipoproteins, smoking, and diabetes. Other factors associated with heart disease include an inactive lifestyle, stress, hormonal factors, and – more important – family history of heart disease, like high blood pressure, diabetes, or even heart attack. This is an over-simplification of the complex laboratory and body characteristics related to heart disease but enough for parents to guide health of growing children.

Over the past four decades, major population studies for heart disease have been conducted worldwide toward understanding these risk factors – especially those that can be controlled. One of the best known studies continues in Framingham, Massachusetts.

Since 1948, residents of that small town near Boston have participated in what is undoubtedly the country's most famous cardiovascular epidemiological or population project. The medical world knows the lives of Framingham residents through an impressive series of bar graphs, bell curves, and trend lines – all representing a "town under the microscope, the home of the 'risk factor.'" My friend Bill Kannel, who directed the Framingham Heart Study for many years, came up with the term "risk factors" in 1961. The BHS is similar in scope but focuses on childhood risk factors, how heart disease begins, and how changes occur into adulthood to study not only heart disease but also aging and longevity.

In Framingham, beginning in the 1950s, Dr. William Kannel described the personal attributes or behaviors that seemed to promote coronary artery disease. Drs. Tom Dawber, Kannel, and William Castelli were pioneers in the field. In 1998, the Boston University Community's weekly newspaper quoted the senior researcher:

"There were cardiologists who felt that obesity and hypertension might be important," says William Kannel, [MD] professor and senior investigator for the Framingham study. "Some felt that diabetes should be looked at. One of our doctors thought that having freckles was a sign that you were predisposed! Almost no one thought that physical activity was good for you. In fact, doctors were advising their patients to avoid it at all costs if they had the slightest suspicion of the presence of heart disease."

My, what has changed! Think of what we have learned.

Today, doctors know that inactivity primes the body for heart failure; they know that high blood pressure and high blood cholesterol increase the likelihood of heart attack; they know that smoking, obesity, and diabetes are all directly linked to incidence of cardiovascular disease. For all those revelations, we can be more indebted to the Framingham study than to any other single source of information about heart health. The Bogalusa Heart Study was so successful in testing children that researchers now have a better understanding of risk factors, and laboratory and medical methods allow studies routinely of children.

Now you can see our advances. Much has been published, debated, and concluded. When researchers conceived the Framingham study, cardiovascular disease was the nation's number one killer. That remains true in the 21st century, throughout the United States and worldwide.

But even 50 years ago, two most famous Boston cardiologists, Paul Dudley White, MD, and Samuel Levine, MD, hypothesized that coronary patients tended to be fatter, have high cholesterol, be diabetic, and smoke. For the first 10 or 12 years, the Framingham study tried to document those associations. News broke in 1961 that cardiovascular risk factors were emerging; the prestigious medical journal *Annals of Internal Medicine* published the story. That announcement changed the medical world but much too slowly. It takes time for the medical community and the public to look at what it takes to be "healthy."

Gradually, physicians everywhere became aware of those patients who showed habitual excesses in eating; whose blood fat levels were elevated; who were obese, sedentary, had high blood pressure, smoked cigarettes; or who exhibited a coronary-prone personality and/or behavior. When these patients were middle-aged men with family histories of heart disease, physicians clearly recognized them as potential heart attack victims. From those days and with new understanding from such studies as described in Chapter Seven, advances have helped sharpen and fine-tune our understanding of lifestyle factors and environment. Medical and surgical advances have helped reduce heart disease and prolong lifespan.

With the discovery of risk factors, medical and public health professionals needed only to inform the populace they could change their behaviors to avoid having heart attacks – *right?*

Wrong, although – and with American Heart Association help – some did. With multiple improvements, understanding, risk factors, and medical and surgical advances, heart disease mortality gradually decreased since the peak around 1965; life span has increased almost 20 years!

To the dismay and chagrin of physicians, most people did not, and still do not, wish to change their behavior – not dramatically or even over the long haul – even when they knew they risked heart disease!

The evolution of reducing risk factors is interesting. Kenneth H. Cooper, MD, and his wife spurred an interest in exercise and gave us the term "aerobics," helping to start the interest in jogging in the United States in the 1960s. Now Dr. Cooper is known internationally as one of the founders of the physical fitness movement that encouraged the growth in the number of joggers from just 100,000 in 1968 to today's 30 million! However, too many people still do not undertake regular exercise, jogging, walking, or otherwise.

Facts became patently clear in another medical study called Multiple Risk Factor Intervention Trial (MRFIT). That study, under sponsorship of the National Heart, Lung, and Blood Institute, tested whether men at high risk for heart disease could reduce their risk factors and also reduce their incidence of illness. Men were selected since they had much more heart attacks than women at a younger age. (That kind of research has changed since it has been realized women have as much heart disease, too, but later in life). Screenings for participants took place in the 1970's. Each of the study's nearly 13,000 men ranging in age from 35 to 57 was screened in 18 cities around the United States. Each participant claimed at least two of the major risk factors: smoking, high blood pressure, obesity, or high levels of blood cholesterol. All said they were motivated to change their lives.

Half of the MRFIT participants knew they were at high risk and went to their personal physicians for the duration of the study. The remainder became a "special intervention" group, who were followed closely, supported, and helped as best anyone knew how to change lifestyles.

When the study ended in 1982, results failed to impress many. Why? One reason: Few failed to change habits, but 40 percent did stop smoking. That was good. But a quirk in the study occurred with excess use of a diuretic; those in the special intervention group under close supervision unexpectedly had more sudden deaths with low potassium (K+). We learned they were given much too much diuretic. We benefitted in that study in helping to understand the use of drugs to treat heart disease and more about arrhythmias (irregular heart beats). We were just learning how to conduct clinical trials.

Part of the problem, we now understand more and more, is heredity. Scientists have shown that the tendency toward obesity and risk factors lies in the genes, not all in the mind or the stomach. Strong evidence points to metabolism – how the body transforms food into energy – as a culprit. Some obese-prone people tend to inherit lower rates of appetite control, or even slower metabolism. Yet, provide the food and calories, and obesity occurs. The problem is complex with hormones or other factors involved. Leptin secreted in the brain turns off appetite, and ghrelins in the stomach adjust dietary intake.

But, even so, naturally slim people enjoy metabolism that adjusts to changes in the number of calories they eat. Just as a thermostat switches on a furnace when a room gets cold, these people have metabolism that revs up to burn off extra calories when they overeat.

The same mechanism can also function in the opposite way. When some people cut calories to lose weight, the metabolic rate slows so that fewer calories are burned for fuel and the *diet* becomes as frustrated as the dieter! From this phenomenon comes the notion of the "yo-yo" syndrome.

Possibly some overweight people have metabolic machinery that fails to switch on at all in the presence of extra calories, making it all too likely that they'll store extra calories as fat. Certain measures of metabolism, such as the rate at which the body consumes oxygen and produces carbon dioxide, can be used to predict who is or is not likely to become obese. Low thyroid function might produce weight gain through accumulation of edema, extra tissue in the body, and slow metabolism. This has to be checked for.

Analyses showed heredity and diet affect even infants. Babies born with even slightly slow metabolism can become overweight by their first birthday! The obese babies in the Bogalusa Heart Study ate no more than the babies of normal weight, but their slower metabolic rate resulted in their piling on extra pounds, and formula feeding fed the problem! Difficulties occur more with bottle-fed infants than those whose mothers breast-feed. Mothers need to understand this observation. Low birthweight (below 5 pounds) from poorer environmental factors during gestation also contributes to a "catch up" and obesity. Unhealthy in utero gestation, especially in the first trimester, from poor diet, alcohol, smoking, affects the developing infant, contributing to later problems. Professor David Barker in England pointed out the long term effect of low birthweight, and we now call it the "Barker hypothesis."

Other theorists look to the brain for fat signals. Understanding of endorphins and other brain chemicals – called neurotransmitters – produced some clues that suggest cravings for certain types of food – fats, carbohydrates or proteins – are governed by neurochemicals. Those foods, in turn, trigger the release of specific brain chemicals, which the individual senses as pleasure. Quite simply, the brain seems to have a sweet tooth *(Mine is for ice cream – oops! I meant to say frozen yogurt.)*

None of these fascinating advances in studying the causes of obesity exonerates other factors, though. The above discussion might be an exaggeration that should not let you, as parents, "off the hook." Strong evidence indicates that environment and lifestyles make a major and significant difference in a child's risk level, even when he or she is born predisposed to obesity with so-called "thrifty" genes. Individuals might have thrifty genes and be healthy but if placed in a different environment or lifestyle, the intrinsic characteristics become expressed to make the individual unhealthy – for example, becoming obese, developing hypertension, or even becoming diabetic.

In this area, diet and a lack of physical activity are prime targets. Only subtle differences might exist between obese and normal-weight children, but small imbalances can lead to obesity. Most kids can become obese by eating as few as 50 extra calories a day (one slice of bread or half a soft drink). That would lead to an excess weight gain of five pounds a year. One soft drink, an extra slice of bread, or half-a-bag of potato chips – that's all it takes! Also consider the availability of food: grocery stores abound and how we do shop – in quantity and now with carts.

Big chain grocery stores make food and all sorts of edible consumer goods irresistible. And how we do fill up those carts! Yet, in low income areas, low-priced food necessitates some folks' buying calorie-dense foods. Note how portion size has increased.

Inactivity comes into play here, with some studies suggesting that the inactivity is a consequence rather than a cause of obesity. *More on obesity and physical activity to follow. . .*

Many or most observers now believe the infiltration of television and computers into the home along with the urbanization of America has contributed significantly to the huge preponderance of obesity that now exists. Kids are bussed to and from school. They ride bicycles less frequently. Playgrounds must have security for use. People simply do not spend as much time engaged in activity, particularly outdoor activity, as before this epidemic of fatness. Here the problem is complex, with social effects on environment.

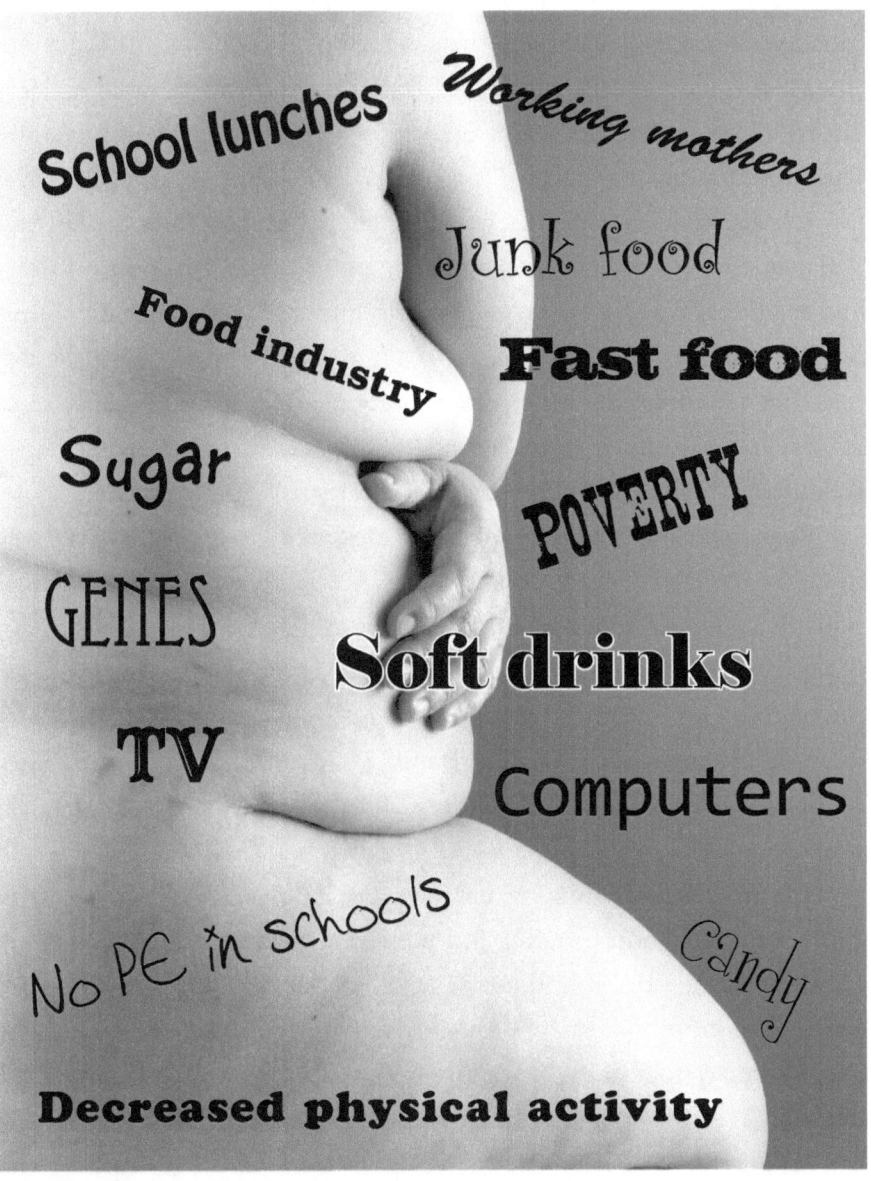

Obesity Epidemic — Complex, Many Contributors

Especially disconcerting is that as weight rises with age, so do the risks of heart disease, diabetes, and stroke. Obesity, measured by skinfold thickness in the BHS, was associated with higher insulin levels and higher blood pressure. This indicated the clustering of multiple cardiovascular disease risk factors, with obesity leading the way. Lean children had less clustering of risk factors than expected, while obese children had more clustering than expected.

Obese children, particularly, get caught in a vicious cycle of rejection and over-eating. As they age, they get swept into a cycle of dieting, losing, and regaining weight. Some people gain and lose a ton over the course of a lifetime!

This yo-yo syndrome prompts people to become metabolically inefficient. With time, the individual requires longer and longer to lose weight and, at the same time, the weight returns faster and faster.

Research suggests the importance of working with body chemistry toward reducing weight to normal levels. Mother Nature tries to help the body defend itself from weight loss; so true and sustained weight loss can occur only when the body can be "tricked" into not going into defense mode. *But, please do not let this be an excuse.*

That genetic-metabolic effect is only a background to the availability of foods – extra calories, calorie-dense foods, empty calories of sugar in drinks.

The way seems simple: eat a good balanced diet of complex carbohydrates, good protein, and poly and mono unsaturated fat – a "healthy eating plan" – and introduce physical activity into every day's routine. Attempt to achieve only needed-calorie intake, energy output, and proper weight gain, especially by children (see growth and BMI charts, pages 36-38.) Reduce saturated fat and refines sugar. This is the argument of obesity occurring in the generation consuming the recommended low-fat diet. Now we are into low carbohydrate diets. For you and your children, learn to choose.

And – *oh, yes!* – another suspected possible contributor to being overweight recently reported could be lack of sleep. National Institutes of Health observations show that infants and toddlers who get less than 12 hours of sleep within each 24-hour span face twice the risk of becoming overweight by age three. Adding two or more hours of television time equates with the risk of body fatness.

Genes plus calories, portion size, metabolism, physical activity, adequate rest – all factor into a child's weight.

Know your numbers and learn what they mean!

Appropriate choices from childhood could have "programmed" you for good heart health — good or bad "numbers." You can assure the same for youngsters you love. You teach, and they will learn healthy decision-making to help improve their "numbers."

We and other research scientists learned lessons that anybody can apply toward improving his or her health and – more importantly – facts on heart risk that can help parents, grandparents, and other adults raise children to be heart-healthy adults.

You can use some of the important "lessons learned" to fix the fat – and also to set and achieve objectives for better heart health! What are the facts?

- The major causes of adult heart disease, atherosclerosis ("hardening of the arteries"), coronary artery disease, and hypertension begin in childhood. Diabetes is closely related to this, while the epidemic of obesity is accelerating these diseases and resulting in adult or type 2 diabetes mellitus in adolescence. We documented changes to the child's cardiovascular system by five to eight years of age, related to the "numbers," the risk factors.

- Heart health risk factors show up early in life, and we have the methods to study heart risk factors. So can your doctor. We have even compared their observations to "normal" values from a large biracial (black/white) population – that is, the Bogalusa

Heart Study. In collaboration, we are comparing findings from the Muscatine, Finnish, and Australian research as described in Chapter Seven. Begin to have your and your family's risk factors determined. Learn the numbers, and know what they mean.

- Ethnic contrasts of risk factors (black/white contrasts) provide underlying clues to how heart diseases occur. We learned from contrasts of black and white individuals living together. Blacks have rampant hypertension, more diabetes, and rampant kidney disease. White men seem to have heart attacks from coronary atherosclerosis earlier. Native Americans have tremendous obesity and diabetes, as much as 80 percent of adult Native Indians. Hispanics tend to be obese and have more diabetes than whites. Japanese, in certain areas of Japan as we mentioned, have the highest stroke rate in the world. Black children and natives in some areas of Tokelauan Islands eating very little salt have little or no hypertension until they move to a Westernized culture in New Zealand. These "experiments in nature" tell us a lot. And all of this can be measured by risk factors. So we repeat: get your numbers and learn what they mean.

- The level of risk factors in childhood differs from those in the adult years. Levels change with growth and different periods of childhood – for example, in the first year of life, during puberty and adolescence, in the transition to young adulthood, and in adulthood. As levels at different ages change an individual, levels can be compared to population studies to get a perspective of being high, low, or normal, again, "percentiles" or the percent, high or low, of the total population.

- Autopsy studies on children and young adults killed accidentally show hardening-artery lesions in the aorta – the largest blood vessel in the body – and coronary vessels, the vessels that circulate on the surface and nourish the heart, later to cause heart attacks. Autopsy studies also show that changes in the kidney blood vessels, as well as those changes in the heart and blood vessels, relate strongly to clinical cardiovascular risk factors, clearly indicating that atherosclerosis, hypertension, and evidence of "adult onset" diabetes begin in childhood. The autopsy findings are the most important observations we have made in the 40 years – underlying cardiovascular lesions in children and adolescents relate strongly to the antemortem (before death) risk factor measured earlier in life. Consider the unbelievable support BHS received from the community to get such information on young people! Distressing – and real.

- Gender and race contrasts contribute significantly to the research findings. As noted previously, African American people experience more severe hypertension; they're diagnosed more with diabetes. *Horrible! All to control in adult clinical medical care.* White males experience early coronary artery disease; white women show a lag in developing coronary artery disease until after menopause. However, smoking and diabetes also contribute to early onset of coronary artery disease in women. Subtle changes of growing up reflect a life-long burden of the cardiovascular risk factors and aging.

- Much of what we consider "environment" relates to behaviors – how we react to the environment and culture. Environmental factors interact with an individual's genetic background and significantly influence risk factors – take dyslipidemia (abnormal lipids or lipoproteins in the blood) as an example: the body's inability to deal with too much fat and sugar in the diet. Hypertension and obesity result from too many calories or too much salt that we cannot avoid. But individuals *can* control environmental factors such as diet, exercise, and cigarette smoking. These are called "modifiable" risk factors; the non-modifiable risk factors include age, race, sex and your family tree. The latter you cannot change.

- Lifestyles and behaviors that influence CV risk are learned and begin early. Individuals must adopt healthy lifestyles in childhood because those healthy habits are critical to changing the risk factors later in life. Primary care physicians, pediatricians, and cardiologists can play a major leadership role in the prevention of adult heart diseases – *beginning in childhood*. Parents, particularly, should ask the family doctor to do "risk factor profiles" on children, along with your "family history" of heart disease, "track" their development, and make recommendations. "Know your numbers" is the start.

Environment often determines lifestyle. For example, if no safe playground is available, after school physical activities might be limited. Available food can be limited by the nature or lack of grocery stores. Distances from medical care can result in lack of medical care. In an area where a lot of adults are smoking, the risk increases for children exposed to tobacco smoke (second-hand smoking) and kids to experiment with tobacco. Adults are the role models.

Now, do you know your own risk factors?

Health-Score Test for youngsters — learning more about health

Life expectancy is not the only consideration for embarking on a healthy lifestyle; your quality of life is equally important.

Take a few minutes to evaluate your child's heart health, and yours. The Health Risk Questionnaire/Heart Score Test which follows can give you an excellent picture of your child's present health and the direction it's headed. For yourself, use the Framingham Heart Study Risk Score Profiles (see http://www.framinghamheartstudy.org/risk/index.html). You can see how well you are now and how healthy your child will be when he or she reaches adulthood. Although you can obtain through different ways several "scores" for adults, the Framingham Study is useful enough and is similar to what insurance companies use for actuarial predictions over the next 10 years.

The test in this book is shorter than the medical questionnaire you fill out in doctors' offices because it deals exclusively with the facts known to impact your child's heart health. Remember that all risk factors link together as if each were tied or tangled with all the others. Look at every factor in your quest for better heart health!

Risk factors interrelate, and obesity centers this relationship. Have one risk factor, such as obesity, and you are likely to have more. Framingham has shown the greater the number of risk factors, the greater the probability of a future heart attack or stroke. Remember, it's like putting money in the bank and allowing it to grow and grow! Controlling risk factors is becoming heart wealthy. Having the burden of risk factors is predictably *disastrous* wealthy.

Now try the following on your kids and see how they are doing.

Answer the following questions as well as you can. To indicate your answer, write the number from the "Possible Score" column in the "Your Score" column that best describes your child. The following numbers are arbitrary but adequate to give you the idea of risk.

Particularly in relation to the BMI and Central Obesity table, the basis for these data is from around 1980, before the epidemic of obesity. Current data after 2000-2005 include children's weight after the obesity epidemic began.

Health Risk Questionnaire/Heart Risk Score

Blood Pressure *In the chart on page 34, Indirect Blood Pressure Measurement By Height, determine your child's height (in centimeters along the bottom) and match it with the blood pressure reading (in numbers along the left side).*	Possible Score	Score
If the higher number of the blood pressure reading (systolic) falls at or above the 90th percentile on the illustration, or the lower number (diastolic) falls at or above the 90th percentile	10	
If the higher number (systolic) falls between the 80th and 90th percentile or the lower number (diastolic) falls between the 80th and 90th percentile	5	
If the higher number (systolic) falls at or below the 80th percentile, and the lower number (diastolic) falls at or below 80th percentile	0	
My Child's Score For This Table		

Body Mass Index & Central Obesity (Abdominal Circumference/Height)	Possible Score	Score
If Body Mass Index (BMI) is above 25	10	
If BMI is between 22 and 25	5	
If BMI is below 22	0	
If abdominal circumference/height is greater than 0.5	5	
My Child's Score For This Table		

Cholesterol	Possible Score	Score
If you do not know your child's cholesterol number	10	
If your child's cholesterol level is 200 or above	10	

If your child's cholesterol level is between 199 and 150	5	
If your child's cholesterol level is 149 or below	0	
My Child's Score For This Table		

Diet — 1 *Select only one of the following three items*	**Possible Score**	**Score**
If your child eats whole milk, ice cream, butter, cheese, bacon, luncheon meats, or fatty meat every day and more than 7 eggs week	8	
If your child eats fatty meat, hamburgers, 4 to 6 times a week, margarine, low-fat dairy products, and 4 to 7 eggs a week	4	
If your child eats poultry, fish, lean red meat, some margarine, skim milk, skim milk products, and fewer than 7 eggs week	0	
My Child's Score For This Table		

Diet — 2 *Select as many of the following as apply*	**Possible Score**	**Score**
If your child snacks on sugary soft drinks, candy, or bakery products daily	5	
If your child eats many salty snacks, such as potato chips, pretzels, crackers, and pickles occasionally	4	
If the person who cooks your child's food uses salt while cooking	4	
If your child salts food at the table	4	
If your child snacks mainly on fruits and vegetables	0	
My Child's Score For This Table		

Exercise	Possible Score	Score
If your child watches TV for long periods, plays computer games, and rarely exercise	10	
If your child exercises, walks briskly, jogs, runs, bicycles or swims for more than 15 minutes less than once a week	5	
If your child exercises that much once or twice a week	3	
If your child exercises that much 3 or 4 times a week	1	
If your child exercises that much 5 times a week or more	0	
My Child's Score For This Table		

Smoking	Possible Score	Score
If your child uses any form of tobacco on a regular basis (once a week or more)	10	
If your child has experimented with cigarettes	2	
If your child has experimented with snuff, pipes, or chewing tobacco	2	
If your child has never tried tobacco	0	
My Child's Score For This Table		

Stress	Possible Score	Score
If your child tends to be very hostile and irritable, overly competitive, and very impatient	6	
If your child is sometimes hostile, irritable, somewhat competitive, a little impatient, and moody	3	
If your child is not hostile, not irritable, not competitive, and usually patient	0	
My Child's Score For This Table		

Family History	Possible Score	Score
If you or any of your child's close blood relatives had a heart attack or stroke before age 60	10	
If any of your child's blood relatives had diabetes at any age	4	
If your child's blood relatives had as a history of high blood pressure	2	
If none of your child's blood relatives had any of the above	0	
My Child's Score For This Table		

Gender *Please check the appropriate box*	Male
	Female

Examination for Heart Disease Risk Factors *Please check the appropriate box*	If your child has **never** been completely **examined** by a physician for heart disease risk factors	Score 5
	If your child has been **completely examined** by a physician for heart disease risk factors	Score 0
My Child's Score For This Table		

My Child's Total Score for Heart Risk	*Total of All Your Child's Scores*

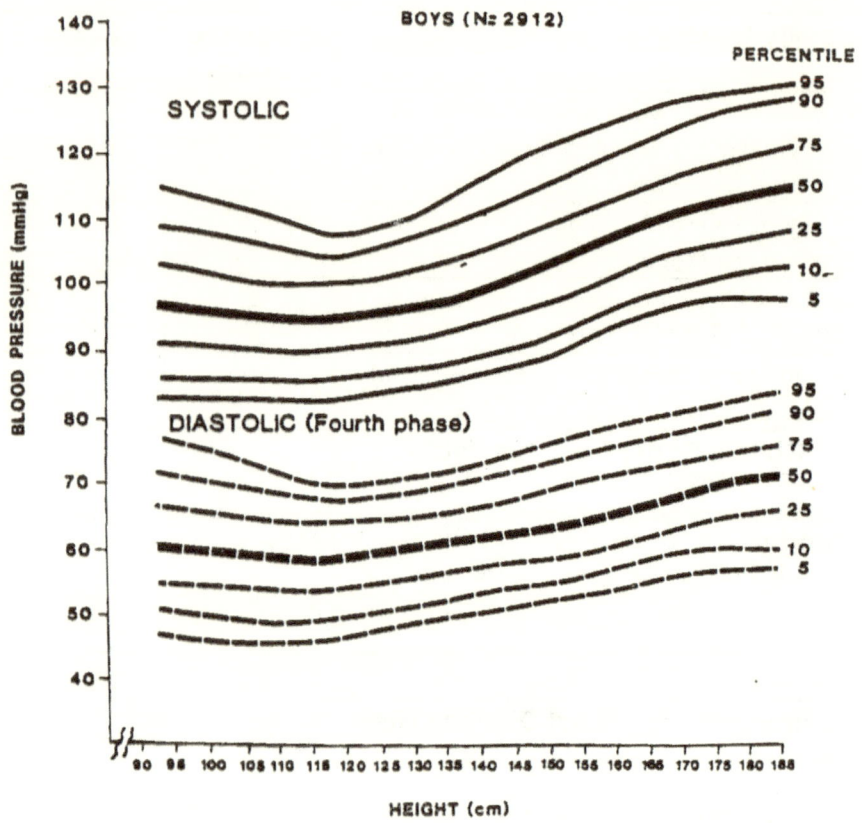

Indirect Blood Pressure Measurement By Height

Do you get the idea?

How worried should you be if your child scored high on this test?

A Heart Risk Score of 36 to 75 is average; so a score of 0 to 35 gives a child an excellent chance of enjoying better-than-average health. A Heart Risk Score of 76 to 110 means that a child's chance – right now – for a healthy future is significantly decreased. *Wow!*

Think about yourself as role model or gatekeeper.

If the score tallies 76 or above, a visit to the family physician should be on your calendar. Please don't delay; now is the time for you and your child to become heart healthy. An average score suggests some important behaviors that should be changed. And a very low score says not only,

"Congratulations!" but also, "Keep it up!" We emphasize "know your numbers" and your child's, too.

If you cannot get your doctor interested, then get another doctor. We consider this stuff seriously.

Your child's total score is the sum of the parts – the individual risk factors, combined. Try the test again a month after completing the book – will you have made progress? Try it on yourself, your spouse, and your children. Please remember that all this scoring is *arbitrary*, but it gives you the idea! The above is just an approximation. Obviously, we don't have an actuarial estimate of lifespan from childhood. Framingham had a lot of data over the 50 years on adults and heart attacks.

Young children develop attitudes and behaviors within the family setting. As they extend their environment beyond the family, behaviors change in response to peer pressure, increasing awareness, and various life influences. Adopting healthy lifestyles leads to good health behavior later and affects health, longevity, and quality of life. At a young age, children can be inoculated against adopting unhealthy lifestyles such as cigarette smoking and illicit drug use while they learn what constitutes a good general lifestyle. Knowing your numbers helps to emphasize prevention.

The following charts, tables, and figures come from the Bogalusa Heart Study. Further levels are available from the Centers for Disease Control and Prevention (CDC), and other resources follow.

Common Percentiles For Height Readings:
The Bogalusa Heart Study

Height by Age:

Males

Age (years)	Percentiles									
	10th		25th		50th		75th		90th	
	Cm	In	Cm	In	Cm	In	Cm	In	Cm	In
5-6	109.8	43.2	113.0	44.5	117.0	46.1	121.1	47.7	125.7	49.5
7-8	120.7	47.5	124.3	48.9	128.4	50.6	133.1	52.4	137.8	54.2
9-10	130.2	51.3	135.4	53.3	139.7	55.0	144.2	56.8	149.3	58.8
11-12	140.1	55.2	144.9	57.1	150.3	59.2	156.7	61.7	164.1	64.6
13-14	153.0	60.2	158.8	62.5	165.0	65.0	170.1	67.0	175.9	69.2
15-16	161.0	63.4	167.4	66.0	172.4	67.9	178.2	70.2	182.2	71.7
17-18	167.8	66.1	171.1	67.4	174.8	68.8	178.7	70.4	182.5	71.8
19-20*	173.0	68.1	174.4	68.7	175.4	69.1	183.5	72.2	190.0	74.8

Females

Age (years)	Percentiles									
	10th		25th		50th		75th		90th	
	Cm	In	Cm	In	Cm	In	Cm	In	Cm	In
5-6	108.8	42.8	112.4	44.2	116.7	45.9	120.3	47.4	124.9	49.2
7-8	119.6	47.1	123.4	48.6	127.6	50.2	131.8	51.9	137.5	54.1
9-10	127.6	50.2	134.3	52.9	140.0	55.1	146.3	57.6	151.7	59.7
11-12	142.3	56.0	148.5	58.5	154.1	60.7	159.1	62.6	162.5	64.0
13-14	151.4	59.6	155.1	61.1	159.6	62.8	163.5	64.4	167.5	65.9
15-16	153.6	60.5	158.3	62.3	161.8	63.7	166.1	65.4	169.9	66.9
17-18	155.2	61.1	158.9	62.6	163.5	64.4	167.4	65.9	172.1	67.8
19-20*	142.9	56.3	150.4	59.2	157.5	62.0	161.2	63.5	167.2	65.8

*Indicates small sample size

Common Percentiles For Weight Readings:
The Bogalusa Heart Study

Weight by Age:

Males

Age (years)	Percentiles									
	10th		25th		50th		75th		90th	
	Kgs	Lbs	Kgs	Lbs	Kgs	Lbs	Kgs	Lbs	Kgs	Lbs
5-6	18.5	40.8	19.5	43.0	21.8	48.0	24.5	54.0	27.5	60.6
7-8	22.3	49.2	24.4	53.8	27.4	60.4	31.4	69.2	37.8	83.3
9-10	27.0	59.5	30.7	67.7	35.9	79.1	43.1	95.0	53.6	118.2
11-12	33.0	72.8	37.2	82.0	44.3	97.7	55.0	121.2	64.8	142.9
13-14	42.5	93.7	48.6	107.1	58.0	127.9	69.9	154.1	82.5	181.9
15-16	50.1	110.4	56.1	123.7	63.7	140.4	74.2	163.6	93.2	205.5
17-18	56.0	123.5	62.6	138.0	73.3	161.6	83.6	184.3	101.1	222.9
19-20*	58.2	128.3	60.1	132.5	76.8	169.3	90.4	199.3	142.2	313.5

Females

Age (years)	Percentiles									
	10th		25th		50th		75th		90th	
	Kgs	Lbs	Kgs	Lbs	Kgs	Lbs	Kgs	Lbs	Kgs	Lbs
5-6	17.1	37.7	19.2	42.3	21.3	47.0	24.1	53.1	27.1	59.7
7-8	21.6	47.6	23.4	51.6	27.3	60.2	33.0	72.8	40.8	89.9
9-10	26.1	57.5	29.7	65.5	36.8	81.1	43.8	96.6	54.0	119.0
11-12	33.5	73.8	40.4	89.1	47.8	105.4	56.4	124.3	68.6	151.2
13-14	42.1	92.8	45.5	100.3	52.4	115.5	64.8	142.9	83.7	184.5
15-16	45.1	99.4	49.5	109.1	58.9	129.8	67.6	149.0	81.1	178.8
17-18	49.1	108.2	52.1	114.9	59.9	132.0	71.3	157.2	95.9	211.4
19-20*	40.7	89.7	59.9	132.1	68.3	150.6	86.9	191.6	94.7	208.8

*Indicates small sample size

Common Percentiles
For Body Mass Index (BMI) Readings:
The Bogalusa Heart Study

BMI (kg/m^2) by Age:

Males

Age (years)	10th	25th	Percentiles 50th	75th	90th
5-6	14.3	15.2	15.9	17.1	18.6
7-8	14.7	15.4	16.5	18.4	21.2
9-10	15.3	16.3	18.1	21.3	25.4
11-12	16.0	17.0	19.1	23.0	26.1
13-14	17.3	18.5	20.8	24.7	29.7
15-16	18.1	19.5	21.2	24.8	31.0
17-18	18.8	21.1	23.7	27.1	32.9
19-20*	19.1	19.7	23.5	29.8	39.4

Females

Age (years)	10th	25th	Percentiles 50th	75th	90th
5-6	13.8	14.6	15.5	17.1	18.5
7-8	14.2	15.2	16.5	19.2	23.0
9-10	14.9	16.3	18.3	21.8	25.2
11-12	16.1	17.2	20.1	23.7	27.2
13-14	17.2	18.5	20.9	24.9	31.1
15-16	17.4	19.0	21.9	25.4	31.4
17-18	18.4	19.8	21.5	26.1	34.4
19-20*	18.3	23.7	26.9	34.5	46.4

*Indicates small sample size

Chapter Four
Obstacles to achieving good health

Every family can *choose* to get healthy – no extra cost, no complicated series of lessons to learn, no extraordinary effort. When adults understand what needs to be done to stay healthy, they can become positive role models to guide their children.

Effective school-based prevention education, like in the Health Ahead/ Heart Smart program (to be described later in this book), promotes health-enhancing behaviors through problem-solving, critical thinking, effective communication, self-initiated learning, and taking responsibility for one's health, beginning in kindergarten. In addition to preparing children to take charge of their own health, we encourage parents and educators to support school children in overcoming social pressures and from participating in violent acts or the use of tobacco, alcohol, or illicit drugs. Early and sustaining efforts of children and youth to adopt healthy lifestyles have the potential lifelong benefit.

You and your family might have devised what you consider a fail-safe plan for achieving good health. But, alas, real life and daily obstacles, both obvious and well-disguised, can intervene and derail the best of plans and intentions. In fact, matters of health get major influence from your heredity, your environment, and your personal behavior.

Obstacle One – Your family tree

If you were a tree, you would be special in terms of leaf shape, bark texture, root depth and breadth, shade- or sun-loving, short and wide, tall and skinny, flexible or unmoving – so many characteristics to consider!

Families come in all shapes and sizes, too. Some are big, others small. Some family members live a long time, others do not. The saying that "the acorn doesn't fall far from the tree" applies to both trees and families. What you inherit from your family can be an important key to the question of who develops heart disease, obesity, diabetes and many other illnesses. No individual can *choose* his or her birth family, but knowing that people inherit characteristics from their parents and grandparents can help youngsters adopt at an early age a lifestyle to minimize risk for these diseases. We encourage in our health education materials that youngsters learn healthy decision-making – getting children early to think good things about themselves. Advances in genetics are slowly, very slowly, helping us understand the influence of genes and the genetic-environmental interaction.

Adults can influence and establish a lifestyle that allows children to avoid risk factors for costly, chronic diseases. Parents, grandparents, and other caregivers should closely monitor a child's lifestyle choices. Who would consciously *choose* to be sick? Does anybody *desire* to be obese or grossly overweight? Who wants to have high blood pressure or high cholesterol? Each, in its own way, can destroy a person's life. And the cost of care skyrockets!

People who have been a part of the BHS since they were children and have been tracked for more than 35 years now comprise an Aging and Longevity Study. As a significant part of the Study, many filled out a total family tree survey, with information on three to four generations of their family to include diseases and ages at death. A family tree is a project you might wish to develop. Include not only parents and grandparents but also blood-related aunts and uncles, siblings, and cousins.

Scientists look at the family tree like a score for the whole family. Some families have many members, including some who die at an early age, and others have people who live a long time with no apparent health problem. The BHS obtained reported parental history of heart attack, high blood pressure, stroke, and sugar diabetes. That history came through as highly significant and related to risk factors of their children. The total family tree can help to focus on future medical problems of the family. We now know subjects in the BHS with little or no risk factors have a family history to include more individuals living above the age of 85 or 90 years. Those with no risk factor had family members living to an older age. *Get the message!*

Anybody who wants to discover the family's roots can use the same family tree package used in the BHS, adapted from studies that Drs. Roger Williams and Steve Hunt began in Utah. They started with school children and with parents and then had them look at family Bibles, visit cemeteries, and talk with many different people to gather the needed information. To complete a detailed family pedigree isn't always easy, but it can be important.

The first page is the basis of the family tree, with information about each person. On another page, individuals record the health of each of their family members: whether they have suffered a heart attack, had a coronary angioplasty (balloon or stent), severe chest pain, high blood pressure, stroke or diabetes, and at what age they experienced these cardiovascular events.

These questions also cover the grandparents and their siblings. Only a small amount of information might relate to the great-grandparents, including whether or not they are still living or, if deceased, at what age they died. Individuals filling out the forms may add things not asked for on the information sheets, including whether they are smokers or non-smokers, since this plays such a large part in the health of an individual.

A family tree data might lack perfection, but beneficial clues will emerge.

Determining the cause or related causes of death for all those grandparents, aunts, and uncles can help you identify potential risk factors for yourself and your children.

My Family Tree

Enter names of family members, relationship, illnesses,
age and cause of death (if deceased), occupation, and
any other information you can gather — try it!

Many resources exist on the Internet to help you construct a family tree.
You can search for and choose from among various "family tree forms."
Several offer free access.
The American Heart Association provides a model at this address:
www.americanheart.org/downloadable/heart.

Obstacles Two and Three: environment and behavior

Environmental and behavioral influences also shape wellness, *big time.* Understanding diet, nutritional habits, and exercise practices of children can help plan treatment strategies or prevention to reduce the natural course of many diseases, such as high blood pressure and diabetes.

Eating a poor diet is a major obstacle. Generally, families who eat nutritious foods, get regular and vigorous exercise, and practice other positive lifestyle behaviors pass these healthy habits on to their children.

The family's environment can affect heart health, too. Fast food restaurants out-advertise and out-sell fresh fruit and vegetable markets. Frequently, fast foods cost less, too. Fewer families today share a scheduled, nutritiously planned and prepared meal – a factor that some experts link to obesity. When is the latest time you sat down with your children, having to eat something you prepared from scratch? A great activity is to involve children in helping prepare foods. Family meals can be a wonderful opportunity for instilling healthy attitudes and values. Help develop young chefs.

Diet is the major environmental factor influencing hypertension. Eating too many calories is clearly related to hypertension; and scientists suggested as early as 1904 that too much salt in the diet is a cause of hypertension. Before the 1970s, the link was established between obesity and high blood pressure in children. High potassium intake has long been recognized to inhibit the development of hypertension. More recent studies suggest that low calcium and magnesium intake, as well as a high ratio of sodium to potassium, are important contributors to hypertension. These minerals are part of a balanced diet. We consume too much sodium (table salt), not enough potassium and magnesium, and often inadequate calcium. After menarche, iron levels in girls might be low. Additionally, polyunsaturated fatty acids and vitamins are implicated in lowering blood pressure (*more on fats and vitamins in Chapter Six.*)

Carbohydrates provide some 48 to 55 percent of a person's energy. Carbs occur in everything – read the labels! The percent of energy contributed by sugar exceeds the recommendation by the United States Department of Agriculture's (USDA) Recommended Daily Allowances (RDA) of less than 10 percent. The percent of energy from protein (about 13 percent) approached the recommended level at all ages, but the percent of energy from total fat exceeds the 30 percent recommendation for infants from six months (35 percent) to four years of age (39 percent). Try to get this down to 25 to 30 percent.

In general, school-age children from 10 to 17 years of age eat the typical American adult diet and also consume a lot of "empty" calories, sugary and salty snack foods, and high fat pizza. Characteristics include a large amount of salt, refined carbohydrates, animal protein, and saturated fat – and low amounts of potassium, complex carbohydrates, vegetable protein, and good fat (more on "good" fat later in this Chapter). Average energy intake ranges from 2,144 calories (age 10) to 2,438 calories (age 17). As expected, boys consume more calories than girls. The USDA recommends that a diet contain no more than 30 percent fat. Yet, fat intake contributes 34 to 38 percent of total calories in children between

10 and 17. Dietary cholesterol intake increases from 302 mg. at age 10 to 378 mg. at age 17 but may exceed 500 mg. The USDA recommendation is to consume one-fourth less. Sodium intake ranges from 3.4 to 3.7 g. in children 10 to 17 years of age. But we don't eat sodium as such; we eat sodium as a salt. Multiply these figures by three so this consists of 12 to 15 gm. of table salt (sodium chloride) and other sodium salts. Half this amount is recommended. Work needs to be done. Salt is ubiquitous, in canned food, in popcorn, in bread and other food items, and as a preservative. Read labels.

Excess caffeine consumption can also pre-dispose youngsters to illness. The caffeine culprits? Regular carbonated beverages, tea, and foods containing chocolate contain caffeine. Caffeine for children can affect blood pressure in negative ways. In the BHS, peak ages of caffeine consumption were two, three, 13 and 17. At age 15, girls begin to consume more caffeine than boys. Yet, for adults, the debate on coffee and caffeine still exists. Although chocolate contains caffeine, the debate on chocolate is being rehashed, and it might not be so bad. *Thanks – but cocoa butter is saturated fat!*

Role models

Parents serve as an important role model for children. The parent who realizes the value of health in his or her own life and who wants to engage in healthy behaviors will be a positive role model. These facts are obvious, so take them to heart.

A parent or other adult role model who avoids smoking, eats nutritious food, exercises regularly, and possesses a healthy and positive self-image will be a more effective health educator than anyone who communicates information and skills without practicing those behaviors. That parent will probably be the most successful candidate in encouraging young children to learn healthy concepts and attitudes and to adopt the necessary skills and behaviors to achieve best health status.

Chapter Five
Your roadmap to better health

Healthy People 2010 asked the United States a valid question: "What are the leading health indicators?"

With 2020 prevention priorities now published, what *do* we have to do to become a healthier nation?

Over three decades, the United States government's Healthy People "framework" has aimed to improve the health of the Nation and individuals by producing public health prevention priorities and actions.

The leading health indicators (LHIs) help measure just how "sound" citizens are. Monitoring those benchmarks for progress encourages collaborations across communities, empowers individuals to make informed health choices, and measures the impact of prevention activities.

This once-a-decade list of prevention priorities covers more factors than the Bogalusa Heart Study considered. *Healthy People 2020* recognizes the import of BHS considerations: "Good nutrition, physical activity, and a healthy body weight are essential parts of a person's overall health and well-being. Together, these can help decrease a person's risk of developing serious health conditions, such as high blood pressure, high cholesterol, diabetes, heart disease, stroke, and cancer. A healthful diet, regular physical activity, and achieving and maintaining a healthy weight also are paramount to managing health conditions so they do not worsen over time."

And more than three decades of evidence from the BHS does provide a roadmap, of sorts, for families who want to be heart-healthy and to grow heart-healthy children. Special areas focus on physical activity, overweight and obesity, tobacco use, and personal responsibility for certain behaviors, particularly having a good attitude.

Complex?

You bet.

Important to know?

Yes – *now more than ever.*

This chapter is longer, more science-oriented, and more difficult than others in the book. But keep reading; think about what you have read; get up and stretch – take a break and return to read. Keep in mind that the facts you are reading about can fundamentally form the methods you use to choose heart-healthy growth for your children. Engage your children in talking about their health and discussing the importance of good decision-making in relation to the family's health. This is your family's health – *It doesn't come in a bottle,* and *you cannot buy it in a drug store or at the supermarket!* You have to work at it. You can earn it.

Essential good behaviors involve nutrition and exercise. Choose low-fat, heart-healthy carbohydrates and adequate good protein of appropriate serving sizes to maintain a healthy weight and avoid obesity. Exercise, exercise, exercise – incorporate cardiovascular and weight-bearing exercises to get and stay fit.

In our follow-up study of children in Bogalusa, some individuals – now 40 to 45 years of age – have developed heart disease and diabetes and are smoking. They were obese in childhood and are still obese. We learned obesity in childhood predicts cardiac enlargement in adulthood and, certainly, high blood pressure and diabetes.

Make sure you and your children eat right, exercise, stay slim, avoid tobacco, and avoid the world's leading cause of death: *heart disease.*

The best good behavior

The best good behavior you can choose and promote is "no tobacco." Tobacco use tops all other preventable causes of premature death in the United States. Every year, more than 400,000 Americans die of tobacco-related disease. Cigarettes cause more than 30 percent of cancer deaths.

Tobacco use remains one of the most important and preventable cardiovascular risk factors. Interest in cigarette smoking includes studying its social and psychological determinants as well as its physiologic consequences. It is addicting.

- Every day some 3,900 youths aged 12-17 try their first cigarette. A few cigarettes and they become addicted. Tobacco is addicting.
- An estimated 6.4 million of today's children can be expected to die prematurely from a smoking-related disease if they continue to smoke at current rates.
- The percentage of high school students who smoke has declined in recent years, but rates remain high: 23 percent of high school students report current cigarette use, this percentage is even higher for white teen girls.
- Fifty-four percent of high school students have tried cigarette smoking.
- Sixteen percent of high school students have smoked a whole cigarette before age 13.
- Nine percent of high school students smoked cigarettes on 20 or more of the past 30 days.
- Eight percent of high school students used smokeless tobacco (14 percent males and two percent females), on one or more of the 30 days before they reported. Adolescents who use smokeless tobacco are more likely than non-users to become cigarette smokers.
- Fourteen percent of high school students smoked cigars, cigarillos, or little cigars on one or more of the 30 days before they reported.
- White boys take on chewing tobacco early.

- Tobacco use may be a prelude to drugs.
- We document <u>consistent</u> smoking in the third grade. The second graders couldn't read the questionnaire!

To examine the influence of cigarette smoking on serum lipid and lipoprotein changes in early life, we re-examined 747 non-smoking nine- to 17-year-olds five to six years after initial screening.

Compared with non-smokers, individuals who begin smoking have more unfavorable changes in serum lipids and lipoprotein levels. These are independent of age, sexual maturation, obesity, alcohol consumption, and oral contraceptive use, which can be related to the lower intensity of early smoking habits. White adults smoking three or more packs of cigarettes weekly show greater increases in very low-density lipoprotein cholesterol, triglycerides, and LDL-C levels. The findings indicate that even modest cigarette smoking starting early has potential long-term cardiovascular risk.

Alcohol usage also has been examined in children and young adults, 12 to 24 years of age. Like cigarette smoking, the prevalence of alcohol consumption increases with age in all race and gender groups. Consistent use, particularly of beer, remains high, even before the legal age to purchase.

Finally, we must factor in exercise and physical activity. The inverse relationship between physical activity and blood pressure is established in adults, but long-term effects of exercise have not been studied in children. Physical activity has a marked effect on the cardiovascular system, with the type of exercise determining cardiac responses in both size and function. In general, exercise might reduce or inhibit hypertension through changes in body weight and body composition.

The BHS – the basis of this book – continues to reveal insight into family lifestyles, choices, and alarming news about obesity, hypertension, tobacco and alcohol use, diet, other disease risk factors, and morbidity and mortality related to cardiovascular disease.

Tobacco links directly to heart disease, stroke, chronic pulmonary disease, and bronchitis. You can stand next to a person who coughs or clears the throat and know that person uses tobacco, probably cigarettes. Oral, tongue, teeth and gum problems, including cancer, often result from chewing tobacco. Notice the round circle of chewing tobacco in the back pocket of blue jeans.

Once addicted to tobacco, any individual faces a life-long battle to beat the behavior of using that killer substance. Yet quitting tobacco diminishes disease risks and can lengthen lifespan. The same applies to alcohol and use of drugs.

Detecting, preventing, and treating risk factors

Studying nearly 2,300 participants in the BHS over two decades showed that children who have very healthy levels of blood sugar, blood pressure, weight, and cholesterol are likely to become heart-healthy adults.

Parents can think of keeping their children healthy as a long-term investment in their lifelong health. Children who are overweight or have high blood pressure are highly likely to carry those problems into adulthood. Cardiac metabolic syndrome (see below, the apple or pear body fat configuration), also known as Syndrome X or insulin resistance, is diagnosed if an individual shows this cluster of risk factors: fat around the waistline, high blood pressure, low levels of high-density lipoprotein (HDL) "good" cholesterol, high fasting blood sugar levels, and high triglycerides. If a person has three or more of these factors, the individual faces higher risk of developing diabetes mellitus and heart disease, as well as kidney disease. The android, masculine, apple configuration or pot belly, the "do lap over," heralds danger ahead.

The *Merriam-Webster Dictionary* describes diabetes mellitus as "a variable disorder of carbohydrate metabolism caused by a combination of hereditary and environmental factors and usually characterized by inadequate secretion or utilization of insulin, by excessive urine production, by excessive amounts of sugar in the blood and urine, and by thirst, hunger, and loss of weight." Such dangers are low, are "silent," however, in childhood. Prediabetes (a poor term recently introduced) also occurs, but it is abnormal. Central obesity (and insulin resistance) and family history are important flags. Besides BMI, measure waist circumference; related to height, it should not be above 0.5.

These results show that the reverse is also true: for the one in 10 children who had very favorable levels of the factors that make up metabolic syndrome, those measures were similarly low in adulthood. Keeping those risk factors low throughout a person's life reduces the risk of various forms of heart disease, many cancers, and other chronic health problems. An additional benefit is reduced health care costs for both children and adults. In our studies in Bogalusa, the one consistent factor in childhood that predicts increased heart size (cardiac enlargement) and thickening of the lining of carotid arteries in the neck in adulthood is obesity – *simply,* obesity!

But what about the children who already face developing diabetes, especially with a family history of diabetes – or those who do not yet experience obesity and can still benefit from prevention?

The Centers for Disease Control and Prevention (CDC) reports that diabetes prevention is proven, possible, and powerful. Studies show that people at high risk for type 2 diabetes can prevent or delay the onset of the disease by losing five to seven percent of their body weight! Eating healthier and getting 30 minutes of physical activity five days a week can be a good start. The prevention-oriented message holds: "small steps that lead to big rewards." A parent's history of adult type 2 diabetes is an awful predictor for children, especially when they become obese. Research shows that Native Americans, Hispanics, and African Americans are at greatest risk.

Obesity's threat

The "very fat" include more males than females and more African Americans than whites, especially females. All face increased risk of cardiovascular disease as they age – and they're likely to die younger than slim counterparts – maybe even at a younger age than their parents.

As an aside to the risk teens are taking in terms of future disease, these overweight and morbidly fat adolescents will also incur higher medical bills. They will require more medical attention, pay more for hypertension and diabetes drugs, likely experience sleep apnea and snoring, and suffer stigma and excess stress.

Scientists – indeed, everyone with access to the Internet – can claim a wealth of knowledge about the lifestyle, dietary habits, and cardiovascular risk factors of people who have participated in the BHS since 1972. Many of those early participants are 40 to 45 years of age now and have children in the Study. What we see in children, we see in parents – *and the reverse!* Very clearly, adult heart disease, hypertension, type 2 diabetes, and obesity begin in childhood and often follow a family pattern.

We know how to study risk factors in children, and we understand that lifestyles begin in childhood. Most of all, we've learned the importance of prevention. As most of the population grows older, study of the aging process and longevity becomes increasingly important from a public health perspective.

Study results prove even more relevant in light of the recent dramatic increase in obesity among youth and adults. While many adults believe that overweight children are simply passing through a harmless phase and will eventually outgrow youthful obesity, research demonstrates a much different conclusion. Many children do not "grow out" of excessive weight gain, especially if they are in families with other hefty eaters and heavy people. Bogalusa researchers have found evidence of coronary heart disease and arteriosclerosis in children as young as five years. Unfortunately, early patterns tend to persist throughout life.

Looking at height and weight, overweight children are going to be obese in adulthood. Risk factors track and are predictive. The message from Bogalusa is that our population is experiencing an epidemic of obesity, an epidemic of coronary artery disease, an epidemic of hypertension, an epidemic of diabetes. The Study also shows that health risk factors often emerge in groups or clusters, leading to more serious chronic diseases later in life.

The RAND Corporation, a non-profit group that addresses challenges facing people around the world, reported that in just five years, from 2000-2005, the United States' obesity rate increased by 24 percent. More disturbing, the increase of severe obesity (greater than the 95th percentile) soared even more.

The National Center for Health Statistics study showed that more than 34 percent of Americans are obese, compared to 32.7 percent who are overweight, with just under six percent classified as "extremely" obese. Two-thirds of all Americans are more than just plain fat!

Similar observations report that fat kids today tend to have the arteries of 45-year-olds and other heart abnormalities that increase risk of heart disease.

Debates continue as to whether obesity is a primary cardiovascular risk factor or whether it influences adult cardiovascular disease through its relationship with serum lipids and lipoproteins and blood pressure levels. Certainly, obesity reflects overall fitness, nutritional status, and activity level. Now we know obesity on its own produces inflammatory, atherogenic factors – *that's dangerous.*

Still, while everybody's talking about appearance – being lean, lithe, svelte, firm, and fit – most Americans fail to achieve it. Obesity, on the other hand, has achieved epidemic status, not only in the United States but on a global stage as well.

The BHS took a look at increasing obesity and "superobesity" (morbid obesity) among youngsters in the early 1980s – two decades *before* most people observed the bulge. Even then, America's children were growing fatter, not fitter. During a two-year period, analysis of 4,223 children showed the prevalence of overweight and obesity; researchers predicted a trend toward what has become a fat nation. Our current data from 2009 in a school-based health clinic shows high school kids are still becoming fatter. The epidemic continues and gets worse.

In general, girls have more body fat than boys. Our children, on average, are 12 pounds heavier, but not taller, than when the Bogalusa research began in the 1970s. The 2009 data suggest 15 to 17 pounds heavier as an average. What was learned in the past few years is that fat around the belly area – central obesity – is a hormonal factory secreting and stimulating inflammatory factors, adipocytokines, which injure the heart and vascular system.

Without behavior change, children with weight problems – even as young as three years of age – likely will struggle the rest of their lives to keep their weight under control. Indeed, studies show that as many as 40 percent become fat adults.

How do you know if your child is overweight? Check the Body Mass Index (BMI) or waist/height values. An early phase that can indicate heart problems to come is this so-called "metabolic syndrome," consisting of the "apple vs. pear" body configuration – apple or android, a man shape with central body fat and belly dropping over his belt is dangerous, and the pear, a nice and feminine, hippy shape less related to early heart disease. The former with central fat disposition is predictive of more cardiovascular disease and diabetes later in life.

The CDC answers many of those "weighty" questions about BMI – including online calculators for both children and adults – on their Website. The calculator for children and teens provides BMI and the corresponding BMI-for-age percentile on a CDC BMI-for-age growth chart. Use this calculator for children and teens, aged two through 19 years. Be careful not to use current levels, but try to use levels established before 1985, before the epidemic of obesity (Look at our tables in Chapter Three.) With the tool, you can provide the child's birth date, the date of having taken height and weight measurements, and the gender. With the answer, you'll learn the percentile in which your child falls and whether that is a heart health risk; if so, the website offers information about what the BMI means and what you can do.

Without access to a calculator, you can divide the child's weight by his or her height squared and, if the measures are in pounds and inches, multiply the result by the conversion factor 703. Or, compare to the tables in Chapter Three. In general, stay under the 85th or 90th percentile, or at or below 25 BMI. Be sure these are age-related. Children's levels of BMI are lower than adults'.

BMI, however, does not perfectly measure body fat, and in some situations the BMI might be misleading. Another useful measure is waist/height ratio, which stays the same as children grow. Get a tape measure. Even with a normal BMI, a waist/height above 0.5 helps relate to central obesity. This value tends to stay constant. If you think your child is overweight, the best idea is to schedule an appointment with your primary care physician or pediatrician to learn the facts. Get a BMI and a waist/height ratio. A cheap way to outguess a CAT scan or MRI – and a tape measure is not nearly as expensive.

The threat of high blood pressure

Hypertension – high blood pressure – is one of the major causes of heart disease. In taking blood pressure, pressure increases when the heart pumps blood into and through vessels in the body. This is systolic or the top (or first) measurement. Blood pressure decreases as the heart relaxes, and the blood flows through the body. This is reported as the low measurement or diastolic phase. We worry about high systolic or diastolic pressure. It is best to check charts for percentiles at a given age or height of a child since blood pressure increases as the child grows (see figure Chapter Three).

For many years, physicians have called hypertension "the silent killer" or "the silent disease" because the person with high blood pressure feels no symptom. The only way to know one's blood pressure is to measure it.

Essential or primary hypertension – that is, without a known or detectable cause – affects one billion people worldwide. Hypertension involves 20 to 40 percent of the United States' population at a relative young adult age and again at early middle age. This high blood pressure is the underlying cause of heart failure, heart enlargement, stroke, kidney disease, and eye problems; and the condition accelerates hardening of arteries, or atherosclerosis and heart attacks. Think of it. Starting at the 85th percentile, cardiac enlargement begins; this is well below what the experts and guidelines recommend.

- Blood pressure tends to increase slightly as the child grows, until about age 14 in girls and 18 in boys. Childhood levels are lower than in adults.
- Hypertension and obesity likely are interrelated, especially in white children.
- Hypertension is more severe and poses a greater chance of illness and death in the black population in the United States, often leading to end stage renal disease, requiring dialysis and transplantation. Hypertension in blacks is a horrible problem.
- Hypertension clusters in families; the presence of hypertension in parents signals a tendency toward the higher blood pressure in a child and later by hypertension.
- Hypertension produces no symptom until heart failure or stroke occurs.

Being overweight and diabetic increases hypertension, and together the two hit the cardiovascular system with a double whammy. Men experience hypertension more frequently than do women. Controlling blood pressure level is as important as to control the glucose level in diabetic individuals.

Secondary hypertension also exists. Usually, secondary hypertension has underlying and detectable causes like kidney disease or is due to a tumor or congenital constriction of the aorta, "coarctation" of the large artery going out of the heart, and coarctation has lower blood pressure in the legs.

Systolic hypertension usually occurs around 40 years of age or earlier. That means the top number – systolic – is high, and the bottom number – diastolic – is normal. An example in an older individual is 160/80. This represents vascular, blood vessel stiffness. But we can observe this vascular stiffness increasing around 25 years of age with our studies of pulses and pulse curves.

In our Westernized, industrial culture, where hypertension is a major cause of heart disease, we eat too much salt, sodium, and not enough potassium. We get most salt as sodium chloride or table salt. But look at labels: sodium bicarbonate, baking powder, bread, cakes, canned foods, even yogurt – all have high salt in them. As stated earlier, we do not get enough potassium, calcium, or magnesium in our diet, and we eat much too much – we take in too many calories. And because most of us do not get enough exercise, we get fat. All this is part of our toxic environment where hypertension occurs in 20 to 40 percent of adults and 60 percent of black adults and maybe 80 to 100 percent in diabetics.

So what can we do? Get your blood pressure taken – taken properly, sitting down, and after resting a few minutes. Make sure the arm cuff is big enough, and have it taken slowly and repeated several times. Ideally, a physician or nurse measures the blood pressure with a sphygmomanometer and a stethoscope over an artery to hear the blood's movement. The observer hears the systolic pressure – the peak of each heartbeat – and the diastolic pressure – by a silence. Now, relatively inexpensive instruments also allow you to take and record your own blood pressure at home; this can be particularly important if you or another person in your home is on treatment for high blood pressure.

Standards for blood pressure readings for adults indicate 130/80 as suspicious of being high, called by the Joint National Commission "pre hypertension." This is a misnomer since any systolic reading above 120 to 125 begins to become elevated in adults. Levels are much lower in children and as with weight stay below the 85th percentile. If weight loss and a healthy diet don't work, seek help from a physician.

Chapter Six
Positive choices pay big rewards

Okay, we have discussed some of the major health problems and learned how to see how unhealthy we are. Now let's get down to doing something about it so that we can become role models for children. We focus on lifestyles and behavior.

Where do you start this life-long process toward fitness instead of fatness and helping both you yourself and your child be heart-smart? Engage the child right now! List the things you know you can do immediately and those you can do as your child grows. Be confident that you can develop and maintain a healthy lifestyle for yourself and your whole family. Share what you read and learn with your youngster at the appropriate age and stage of growth. Are your children getting health messages at school, from their friends, or from watching TV? Check it out by asking them. Talk to your kids about what they eat that you don't know about and explore physical activity, smoking, and other children's activities.

What is health? Simply not being sick, having a sound body, mind, and soul, having a sense of well-being – all these and other values appear in published and generally understood definitions of the word "health."

Researchers at the BHS found that lifestyles and behaviors which influence health are learned and begin early in life. Therefore, common sense suggests that healthy lifestyles should be adopted in early childhood. Changing behavior is much more difficult later in life. Primary care physicians, pediatricians, and cardiologists can play major leadership roles in the prevention of diseases beginning in childhood. But parents, grandparents, or nannies of small children have the most important role to play in the young child's development.

So where do you begin? *Healthy People 2020* – the nation's "framework for prevention" – offers Leading Health Indicators, selected on the basis of their ability to motivate action, the availability of data to measure progress, and their importance as public health issues. Twenty-six indicators are organized under 12 topics:

- Physical activity
- Overweight and obesity
- Tobacco use
- Substance abuse
- Responsible sexual behavior
- Mental health
- Injury and violence
- Environmental quality
- Immunization
- Access to health care

Obviously, all this is not under our scope, but much is.

Our Health Ahead/Heart Smart curriculum adds to these, beginning in kindergarten health education – K-3 lesson plans, called "It's Me." In addition to emphasizing the three magic words – "please, thank you" – we discuss respect, compassion, ethics, morals, and healthy attitudes (See Appendix.)

The American Heart Association says that a healthy diet and lifestyle can be the "best weapons" to fighting disease – how much better to choose good nutrition and lifestyle paths *before* having to combat illness.

While nutrition science continues to evolve with new findings from research, we have no such thing as an "ideal" diet. Most dietitians and other health advocates recommend similar strategies:

- Eat a healthy breakfast and other meals at appropriate intervals;

never allow yourself to get so hungry that you over-eat when you do stop for a meal. Some people actually function better with multiple mini-meals throughout the day, and this tends to be healthier without big spurts of blood glucose and insulin.

- Monitor portions and calories as well as the macronutrients, the fat, protein and carbohydrate mix; the United States Department of Agriculture suggests that approximately 50 percent of calories should come from carefully chosen carbohydrates, about 30 percent from fats, and approximately 20 percent from protein sources.

- Snack, but little on "junk" food – select no-fat, low-sugar, high-fiber, complex carbohydrates such as fruits and vegetables. The farther away from the "farm" or garden, and the closer to processed food, the more unhealthy.

- Exercise regularly, *more on this subject later.*

- Sleep appropriately for your age and stage in life. The Centers for Disease Control and Prevention recommends adults get seven to nine hours, adolescents from 7.5 to 9.5 hours, and varying intervals for babies, toddlers, and young children – from 18 hours for newborns to nine to 11 hours for children aged five to 12.

- Eliminate tobacco products – no smoking, chewing, or dipping snuff! These should not have started, but nip the bud by kids' experimenting.

- Maintain a moderate weight. Balance calories by weighing frequently and at a constant time, like upon waking up in the morning.

- Drink alcohol *only* in moderation, as adults. This is not in the culture of children, but be open about it.

Achieving good health from the start

Research underscores the role that lifestyle and behavior, such as poor diet and inactivity, play in disease. Adopted within a child's first few years of life, parental choices dramatically influence cardiovascular risk later on.

The answer lies in early intervention and prevention.

As we wrote in the latest of five textbooks based on BHS observations, adverse cardiovascular risk factors start early in life. The most dramatic evidence comes from autopsy studies on young individuals in Bogalusa.

From our autopsy studies, we note that virtually 90 percent of our population by the third decade of their lives have early evidence of atherosclerosis. An autopsy study was done on Korean and Vietnam War soldiers. Some 70 percent of the soldiers, who would have been about 22 years, had significant coronary artery disease. This is what we found in our Bogalusa autopsy studies, and it is also what they find in the Pathologic Determinants of Atherosclerosis in Youth (PDAY) study, which is a multicenter study of autopsies of 15- to 35-year-old individuals. This is universal across a Westernized population. Germany, England, Switzerland, and other countries all have similar changes.

The obesity epidemic contributes to hypertension and diabetes and is accelerating the level of atherosclerosis. Obesity certainly has accelerated diabetes and diabetes coupled with other risk factors that relate strongly to vascular disease and coronary artery disease.

The best approach for preventing heart disease and diabetes from developing in adults – both blacks and whites – is early diagnosis. Individuals must remind their physicians to look at coronary artery disease in early life and to emphasize prevention all along the way. This is really the physician's role: to lead public health education in the school system and develop prevention strategies for families and children.

We strongly encourage what is known as "primordial prevention," which is to treat risk factors as they begin. The best place to start primordial prevention is in the schools system, where it's easy to get height, weight, and blood pressure as well as to check for vaccinations. We have the materials (see Appendix); we know how to use them; and we know it works. We have seen one school in Louisiana where 20 of 120 children actually lost weight. The average weight gain for growing children in that school would have been five pounds, and it fell to 1.7 pounds. We are helping with a multi-practice clinic that has a grant to work with children at the 95th percentile of obesity. The children are bussed in, taught about nutrition, given an exercise program, and they lose weight and are doing great. Parents are involved.

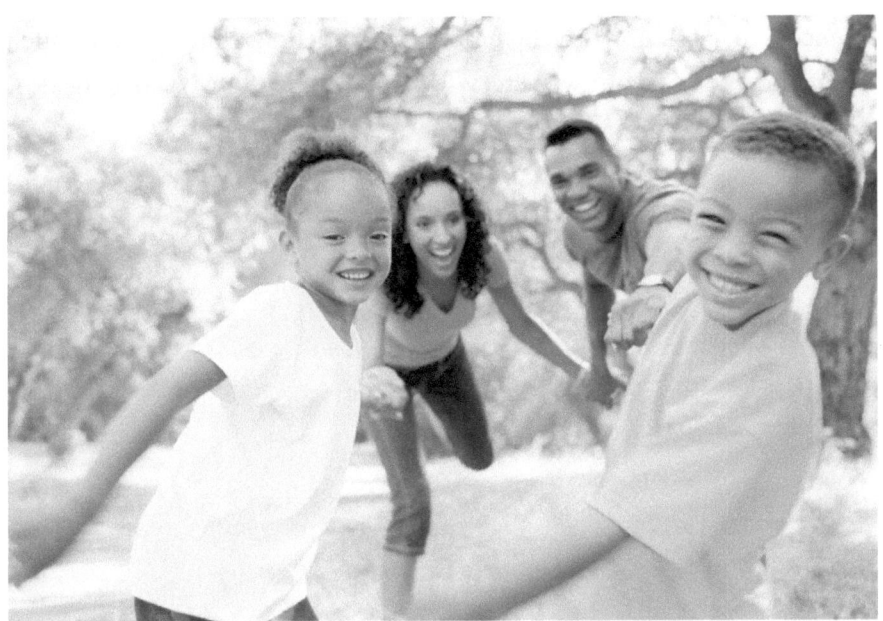

Growing Up Fit

Parental choices about lifestyle and behavior
dramatically influence cardiovascular risk for the whole family.

Aim for these positive actions & attitudes

Live Longer – Healthy	Much More Exercise
Smiles – A Good Attitude	Less Fat
Enjoy Life With Health	More Fiber
Smart Eating = Fun	Less Alcohol
Enrich Your Child's Life	More Fruits & Veggies

We ought to be doing this in schools everywhere, but it is not yet happening. It took 40 years for the consumer public to accept the effects of smoking on lung cancer and heart disease; so if we'd had the first data on risk factors in children 20 years ago, we might still have about another 20 years to go before this concept is accepted. Can we afford to wait for you and your kids? The American Heart Association presented new guidelines for screening at the 2011 meeting; so maybe eventually our science will catch up with the practices. Guidelines don't tell too much about "how to." See our website, www.Tulane.edu/SOM/Cardiohealth.

Chapter Seven
Feasting on nutritious food – *or not*

I am what I eat – really! With so many suggestions, cookbooks, and nutrition experts, what's real?

Most health and nutrition experts suggest a diet with less than 7 to 10 percent of calories from saturated fat and no more than 30 percent of calories from total fat. To achieve this, food choices should include more plant foods – vegetables, fruits, grains – with little, if any, added fat. Low-fat dairy products, fish, and very lean meat and poultry can be included, too. Try a home-cooked meal with family.

The following are a few specific recommendations to begin a more nutritious lifestyle.

Eat at least five servings of fruits and vegetables daily. Fruits and vegetables can fill you up and provide needed vitamins, minerals, antioxidants, and fiber. Nutritionists, educators, and researchers associated with the BHS, especially Theresa Nicklas, DrPH, LDN, designed "Gimme 5," a health promotion effort to learn to eat five servings of fruits and vegetables a day. Here are just a few ways to accomplish this goal:

- Eat a banana with cereal, or strawberries, or fresh peach.
- Have a salad with fresh ingredients and low- or no-fat dressing for lunch.
- Eat an apple, a pear, or some plums as a snack.
- Enjoy a fruit salad in mid-afternoon.

- Steam some vegetables for dinner.
- Snack on fruit and low-fat cheese or prepared munchies such as mini-carrots, celery; you can add a few unsalted nuts, preferably walnuts or almonds.
- Have fun making a smoothie with vegetables and fruits added to yogurt and low- or no-fat milk.

Try a Mediterranean diet, but not with excess calories!

A research program funded by the National Institutes of Health (NIH) developed a healthy lifestyle plan based on the Dietary Approaches to Stop Hypertension (DASH) diet (based on the Mediterranean Diet). It helped to lower blood pressure without medication. The DASH Diet Action Plan provides a complete lifestyle program to support reaching and maintaining a healthy weight and to lower blood pressure and cholesterol.

The DASH nutrition plan recommends:

- More grains and grain products than any other food group.
- Plenty of fruits and vegetables.
- Low- or non-fat dairy products.
- Larger amount of fish, even fatty fish, less farm-raised, with some amounts of lean poultry and meats.
- Very limited quantities of fats and sweets.
- Peas, beans, seeds, and/or nuts.
- Substitution of olive oil for saturated fats, such as butter or lard.

We add these:

- Trim the fat.
- Hold the salt.
- Reduce the sugar.
- Broil, bake. Reduce frying but do with olive oil or polyunsaturates, like Canola.
- Read labels.

- Watch the calories, the calories, the calories.

Reduce foods containing saturated fats – *more on fats later in this chapter.*

To achieve a diet with less than 10 percent of calories from saturated fat and no more than 30 percent of calories from total fat, food choices should include more foods from plants – vegetables, fruits, grains – with little, if any, added fat. Low-fat dairy products, fish, and lean meat and poultry can be included. The authors of *Healthy People 2010* state, "Persons in the United States consume too much dietary fat in general, and too much of the fat consumed is from saturated fatty acids – the type associated with an increased risk for heart disease."

Exercise portion control. Within just a few years, the food service industry has increased portion sizes by up to 25 percent! Notice the size of hamburgers being advertised in fast food outlets. So what do most nutritionists consider to be a "normal" serving size? You can use your hand, visual imagery, or actual measuring tools (spoons, cups, a food scale, or size of plates) to estimate the number of calories to be eaten.

A word about fat in your diet: Fat and maybe refined sugar impact cholesterol levels in the blood more than cholesterol in food. Low-density lipoproteins – the special carriers of cholesterol in the blood – carry cholesterol to the arteries, while high-density lipoproteins carry cholesterol to the liver to be excreted. Not all fats carry cholesterol in the same way.

Three types of dietary fat affect cholesterol differently: saturated, polyunsaturated, and monosaturated. The latter two have considerable variations in the different oils – palm has a lot of saturated, olive oil monounsaturated, and canola, corn, and soy have polyunsaturated. Oily fish from northern waters and not farm-raised have the healthy omega 3 fatty acids that affect cell membranes and help lower triglycerides.

The fact is, however, that **nobody has an ideal diet**, even though researchers are improving recommendations all the time. Experts in the field simply recommend a balanced diet with ideal caloric needs and some modification only for children with certain diseases. Be calorie-conscious!

Dietary intake is only one aspect of lifestyles and behaviors that forms a basis for healthy living and children's growing up healthy. With our modern style of living, we must also recognize physical activity and exercise as equally and critically important lifestyle components. We must prevent bad habits – like smoking cigarettes, completely avoidable and unnecessary.

Far too few of the weight-loss writers can prove any success – especially toward long-term weight loss and health improvement – beyond lowering the bank accounts of book-buyers by the horde looking for a fast fix. And, still, the epidemic of obesity in children and adults continues and escalates. Two-thirds of the United States' population is obese, and one-third of all children have surpassed fatness to obesity. Poor lifestyles continue to run rampant.

Fat is a fact. So are sugar, calories, and salt. And the facts should scare every obese person into looking beyond the physical attribute and its damage and danger to the body – in almost-sure-to-follow harm from hypertension, high cholesterol, diabetes, and deadly heart disease.

Finally, emerging research shows that having "family meals" can be healthier for every member of the family. Doesn't your family deserve that treat to stop everything and sit down to eat together? Make it a time to relax, communicate about what's happening in your various lives, and share new experiences. Eat together! Let children help plan meals and start their learning from a young but safe age how to prepare nutritious foods. Experiment with foods from different cultures, talk about and practice polite table manners, have fun! And enjoy the knowledge that if you've planned, purchased, and prepared fresh fruits and vegetables, you've probably saved some money, too!

Using nutritional Information

Following a meeting on nutrition at a New Orleans school, a young mother stayed on to talk about the problem of heart disease in children. She was glad to learn more about cholesterol, especially because her own two children had tested in a high range. She was determined to try to serve healthier foods to her family: low-fat milk (preferably fat-free) instead of whole milk, fish more often, fresh fruits, vegetables, and lean meats.

As she turned to leave, she said, "And what has made it even easier is that my kids just love peanut butter, which has zero cholesterol. Between them, they can polish off a jar in the course of an afternoon!" *Wow.*

Beware: peanut butter is loaded with salt and high-energy, calorie-dense oil. If peanut butter is a choice, use natural peanut butter which is not hydrogenated and contains less harmful fat; this often separates and must be mixed before serving.

That mother is not the only person with a misconception about cholesterol, oils, and food labels. Shoppers search supermarket shelves for foods labeled "cholesterol-free," assuming that such foods are healthy. Too few consumers actually know what cholesterol is and how it can help or harm the body's health. The National Institutes of Health describes cholesterol as "a waxy, fat-like substance that occurs naturally in all parts of the body" and says: "Your body needs some cholesterol to work properly. But if you have too much in your blood, it can stick to the walls of your arteries. This is called plaque. Plaque can narrow your arteries or even block them. High levels of cholesterol in the blood can increase your risk of heart disease. Your cholesterol levels tend to rise as you get older. There are usually no signs or symptoms that you have high blood cholesterol, but it can be detected with a blood test. You are likely to have high cholesterol if members of your family have it, if you are overweight or if you eat a lot of fatty foods."

Remember the admonition about throwing mud at the barn door; some eventually sticks. Keep up bad lifestyles and poor diets to see what harm can occur.

And also remember that hypertension is a "silent" disease; get your blood pressure checked!

Cholesterol comes from food and what the body produces – primarily by the liver and other cells. Vegetables and fruits do not contain cholesterol, but animal products and fish do. A plant-based diet is low cholesterol and low fat.

Unfortunately, some "cholesterol-free" foods actually contain more fat than a lean steak. Other shoppers opt for "low-fat," two-percent-fat milk, thinking – *mistakenly* – that is a big improvement over whole milk. Two-percent-fat milk has 20 times more fat than skim milk. Still more choose "health foods," assuming all items so marked are good for the heart. Ads can be catchy and misleading! They're designed to sell. Their common mistake is that cholesterol is the only ingredient to avoid when, actually, the other major villains are saturated fat, transfat (from hydrogenation), excess sodium, and simple sugars, sucrose, and cornstarch. The greater trend of cornstarch use has paralleled the epidemic of obesity.

Too much of all fat can harm because it is high in calories and enhances forming abnormal lipoproteins. Fat supplies nine calories per gram – more than twice as many as protein or carbohydrate, each of which supplies four calories per gram. So even if doing no other harm, consuming fat can make a person overweight.

Avoid saturated fat!

Saturated fats stay solid at room temperature. Good examples are lard, Crisco®, and other hydrogenated vegetable oils. Mainly from animal sources, these fats are in meat and whole-milk products. The breast of poultry and fish contain some saturated fat but usually less than in beef, pork, and other meat. Skinned chicken or turkey breast can considerably reduce fat. Processed meats are worse, being high in fat and salt.

When buying hamburger meat, limit the fat to no more than seven percent. Selected cuts of meat, when ground, can get to as little as three percent. Before using hamburger meat to cook foods such as chili, spaghetti sauce, and tacos, drain the cooked beef in a colander lined with a paper towel. To eliminate even more fat, rinse the drained beef under HOT water before placing it back in the pot. To really lower fat in ground beef, heat in a skillet with a polyunsaturated oil like soy or canola and then pour off all the oil.

Three types of vegetable oils are high in saturated fat – palm, palm kernel, and coconut. Palm is cheap and often used. Read the labels. Although print says "contains no cholesterol," one tablespoon of palm kernel oil or coconut oil contains more saturated fat than an equal amount of butter or lard. These oils are in cake mixes, non-dairy creamers, solid vegetable shortenings, and chocolate candy. Why do manufacturers continue to put these unhealthy oils in products we buy? Because they cost less and have a longer shelf-life.

Here is an interesting side note: a research team at the University of Texas found that the fat in beef and chocolate is not quite as "bad" as originally believed. In fact, such fat showed a tendency to lower cholesterol levels. Before millions of Americans could dash away to a dinner of steak and chocolate fudge cake, however, the researchers added that these foods also contain other fats known to raise cholesterol levels – namely, palm and coconut oils often used in pastry. This area is still in limbo; so the best advice about this problem is to eat these foods in moderation.

To be sure, however, saturated fats raise the levels of both the good, high-density, and bad, low-density, lipoproteins in the blood, particularly when mixed with high refined sugar. This is what gets deposited in the artery wall.

Research suggests the possibility that people can be fat-sensitive or non-fat-sensitive. Those who "do well" or find their cholesterol levels dropping while they are on cholesterol- or fat-restricted diets probably benefit more from reducing saturated fat, according to a research team at the University of Texas Southwestern Medical Center in Dallas. Here, heredity and metabolic differences may play a role. When we fed monkeys a high fat-cholesterol diet, some responded more, some much less. Those developing high cholesterol levels, we called "responders," others "non responders." That, for experimenting, is close to humans.

Liquid at room temperature, **polyunsaturated fats** come from plant sources and are found in cooking oils, margarines, and many salad dressings. Even among the polyunsaturates, a hierarchy exists of those considered better or worse: canola, safflower, sunflower, corn, sesame, and soybean oils are recommended because they are lowest in saturated fat and highest in polyunsaturated fat. Cottonseed oil and generic vegetable oil are at the bottom of the list because they have more saturated fat. Polyunsaturated fats lower cholesterol, including both high-density lipoproteins and low-density lipoproteins. The body cannot make the double bonds found in chemistry of polyunsaturated and monounsaturated fat, and they are referred to as essential fatty acids.

A common question surfaces: "If polyunsaturated fats are always liquid, what about margarines, which are supposed to be polyunsaturated?"

Oils in solid shortening and margarine are partially hydrogenated to make them firmer and to have a better shelf life. During the hydrogenation process, oils become more saturated. Also, with hydrogenation the structure is twisted to become trans, which attack the body like saturated fat. The temperature used to cook determines the breakdown of essential fatty acids, so limit frying and high temperatures.

Also liquid at room temperature, **monosaturated fats** come from plant sources such as avocados, peanuts, and olives. Research suggests that monosaturated fats – especially olive oil – lower only the low-density lipoproteins. Olive oil is the major oil in the Mediterranean countries and a big part of the Mediterranean diet.

Wise choices in the supermarket

- Whenever possible, select the white meat of chicken and turkey for lowest fat meat.
- Limit the skin of poultry.
- Do not buy and do not deep-fry foods.

- Whenever possible, chose fresh and frozen foods rather than canned, high- salt. Commercial foods in cans are high in salt.
- Whole grain bread and cereals are the best choices.
- Try to eat at least five servings of fruit and vegetables every day.
- Above all, watch calories.

So, what do you put on your toast?

With a huge array of products in the supermarket's dairy section, all the facts you've learned can be easily forgotten, leaving you with nothing but labels to make your decision. Should you choose soft margarine in tubs, in squeeze bottles, in sticks, a margarine-butter blend, margarine substitutes, or – *finally!* – regular butter? Keep it simple, weigh in the calories.

- A tablespoon of stick margarine has about 100 calories, 11 grams of fat, 2 grams of saturated fat and no cholesterol. Squeeze and tub margarines are less hydrogenated than other forms and, therefore, are higher in polyunsaturated fats and a better choice.
- Diet margarines have 50 calories, 6 grams of fat, 1 gram of saturated fat, and no cholesterol per tablespoon. Margarine-butter blends contain from 90 to 100 calories, about 10 grams of fat, 3 grams of saturated fat, and between 5 and 10 mg of cholesterol per tablespoon. The more solid, the more hydrogenated, the more saturated and trans. Tend to skip.
- Butter has about 100 calories, 11 grams of fat, 7 grams of saturated fat, and 31 milligrams of cholesterol per tablespoon! If you stick with butter, use in limited amounts and infrequently. Julia Child would disagree, since butter surely makes food taste better. *Sorry!* Butter surely helped raise the serum cholesterol in our monkeys.

But what about the bread – the toast, crackers, muffins, and bagels that attract the popular spreads? Here's a rundown:

- Crackers – depends entirely on the brand and type, with no-fat, low-sodium saltines providing 32 mg sodium and 4 g carbohydrates. You can compare them in terms of calories and fat content. Read the labels.
- Wheat bran muffins – 112 calories, 3 grams of fat, 1 gram saturated fat, 0 cholesterol.
- Corn muffins – prepared from dry mix, 91 calories with 26 from fat, 3 g fat, 18 mg cholesterol, and 222 mg sodium.
- Plain two-and-a-half-inch bagel – 72 calories, 0 grams of fat, 139 mg sodium and 14 g of carbohydrates. Note: my bagels tend to be bigger.
- White bread – refined wheat flour loses fiber and needs added vitamins.
- Whole wheat bagel – from 120 to 360 calories (depending on the manufacturer), at least 1 gram of fat, 0 saturated fat, 0 cholesterol, and 270 to 620 mg sodium.
- Oat grain and soluble fiber are your best choices – here, we are comparing and just showing variations.
- English muffins vary by maker. Read the labels.

This begins to reveal why Americans get 15 percent of their fat from breads and cereals. In summary, here are some tips for you – remember:

- Populations on diets low in saturated fatty acids and cholesterol experience low risks and rates of disease. Most of the saturated fat a person eats comes from meats and dairy products; simply choosing nonfat or low-fat dairy products and lean meat should reduce risk. Cheese is usually high fat; note the kind of milk used for preparation. The best choices for fat in the diet – and everybody needs *some* fat – come from mono and polyunsaturated fatty acids such as in olive, safflower, sunflower, and canola oils – and from a few nuts (almonds and walnuts, for example).
- Food labels can confuse! The bottom line and most important

factor to remember is this: people must reduce both fat and dietary cholesterol in the food they eat, especially saturated fat, and aim to achieve an ideal body weight.

- Approximately 25 to 30 percent of all children from age 5 to 18 have excessive levels of cholesterol in their blood, which means they are at risk for serious disease as adults.

How can you make your diet healthier?

- Substitute polyunsaturated fat for saturated fats whenever possible.
- If you must use salt, use less. You might prefer a salt substitute.
- Sugar – you need some sugar? Try fruit as a good choice.
- Peanut butter – choose natural; read the label; stay within the limits.
- Chips – you certainly may eat potato chips, just not often.
- Donuts – yes, some, but only occasionally.
- Ice Cream? Try frozen yogurt instead.

Vignettes and references

We can be grateful to the pioneers who studied various aspects of coronary heart disease, especially beginning in the 1940's and 1950's, and who helped us begin to know that diet and lifestyles do affect our heart health.

- Taking these lessons and urging by the American Heart Association led the number of deaths from heart disease to begin dropping from the high around 1965. Finland, with the highest heart disease rate in the world, took hold around 1975 with the **North Karelia Project**, spearheaded by Pekka Puska, MD, who became director of the National Health Institute of Finland in 2003. Incidentally, Dr. Puska contributed to our Family Health Promotion program; see http://tulane.edu/som/cardiohealth/family.cfm. Finland drastically reduced heart attacks by reducing smoking and reducing saturated fat in the diet. This study report appears on the website http://www.cvhpinstitute.org/links/northk.htm.

- **The Seven Countries Study** by Ancel Keys, PhD, and carried on by a friend, Henry Blackburn, Europe and United States, showed cultural differences like dietary intake of fat and cholesterol related to marked differences in serum cholesterol level and mortality. Southern Italy and Greece have longer life spans and significant cultural differences, lower fat and cholesterol intake, and lower blood cholesterol levels – so much so that a famous United States epidemiologist *bought villas* on the Mediterranean coast.

- The **Japanese, Honolulu, San Francisco (NiHonSan) Study** with migration patterns of Japanese, while carrying the same gene pool, showed that the closer to the United States, the more heart disease and diabetes occurred. The current trends and adoption of Westernized culture in Japan has now affected the children with obesity and cholesterol levels higher than their parents'. Rickshaws have disappeared. This is another "experiment in nature" that shows the importance of environment.

- Tulane University physician and educator Timothy Harlan, MD, also known as "**Dr. Gourmet**," maintains a Website, www.drgourmet.com, that offers healthy recipes and meal plans related to the Mediterranean-style diet. Yet, Martyn Katan, MD, showed a Mediterranean diet can be atherogenic with increasing calories and obesity. The message: *watch calories and weigh often.*

- Still another resource on **nutrition basics** and how to control fat consumption while eating appropriate carbohydrates and protein comes from the Centers for Disease Control and Prevention (CDC): www.cdc.gov/nccdphp/dnpa/nutrition/nutrition_for_everyone/basics.

- **Frank Sacks**, MD, at Harvard studied four different styles of diets, very low in saturated fat, high fat, low, and high carbohydrate. If subjects lost weight, blood lipid patterns showed no difference.

- **Framingham Heart Study** – William B. Kannel, MD, MPH, and his senior colleague – Thomas R. Dawber, MD, director of the Framingham Study from 1949 through 1966. Kannel joined the study in1949 and directed the project from 1966 to 1979. William P. Castelli, MD, became director of the study in 1979, a role he retained until 1995, when Dan Levy, MD, took over as the fourth director. They led the way. Use the Framingham Score (http://www.framinghamheartstudy.org/risk/index.html) for a rough index of your own cardiovascular score.

Chapter Eight
Kid Fit:
Engage and enjoy physical activity

Lime green rubber boots with frog faces on the toes made scrunch noises on the floor as Josh ran through the kitchen. He grabbed his favorite blue denim hat off the rack, pulled it over his uncombed brown hair, and dashed out the door.

"Joshua," his mother called his full name to get his immediate attention. "Stop this minute. Where are you going?"

"I've got to help Dad wash the car," the youngster said. "I'm a big boy now and I've got to help Dad."

Josh's mom, Sandy, smiled to herself and felt pleased that Josh still wanted to run, play, and help his dad instead of watching cartoons on television or playing with games in his room.

Sandy recalled her own mother's counsel: "We've got to practice good health behaviors ourselves so we all can avoid joining the fast-growing fat folks' society! That's so important to being healthy – keeping a normal weight, getting exercise, avoiding tobacco and drugs, and keeping a positive attitude."

The national focus on early childhood education *must* begin with the health of every child. This includes being well-nourished, activity-oriented, and prepared to learn. The key to developing such children starts in the home and involves the whole community in which children can grow and thrive.

But a government-funded study in early 2009 reported grim news on obesity: the number of obese American adults for the first time outweighs the number of those who are considered merely overweight. The National Center for Health Statistics study showed that more than 34 percent of Americans are obese compared to 32.7 percent who are overweight, with six percent classified as "extremely" obese. Two-thirds of all Americans are more than just fat! Is bariatric surgery the answer? *Certainly not for the majority of the population.*

An April 2008 news report from MSNBC said, "Some experts say we as a nation are doing ourselves in with our couch-potato culture of eating way too much and exercising far too little. Some health professionals even raise the controversial notion that today's generation of kids – about a third of whom are overweight or obese – might be the first to live shorter lives than their parents."

Children and teens need 60 minutes of physical activity every day and adults 18 and older at least 30 minutes every five of seven days to be and stay healthy – that according to The President's Council on Physical Fitness and Sports.

The Council reported that including a 30-minute brisk walk or leaf-raking, 15 –minute run, or 45-minute volleyball game can give significant health benefits. Equally good news, the more the activity, the better the results. Just look at body structure, and you can guess what type exercise — weight vs. jogging, or none.

How to reduce the risk of developing or dying from cardiovascular disease, type 2 diabetes, and some cancers – how to lower blood pressure and cholesterol, prevent or slow osteoporosis, lose weight (aka "fix the fat") and reduce the symptoms of arthritis, anxiety, and depression? Engage in even moderate daily physical activity. Find physical activity you enjoy and have fun!

Exercise offers more benefit than just controlling calories. For yourself, consider preventing osteoporosis or helping reduce stress, anxiety, and depression. Just remember that exercise is not a cure-all and that extreme or stressful exercise can result in injuries.

Based on the prevalence of obesity and other health-related statistics, most people fail to get enough exercise. People who do not engage in physical activity are twice as likely to suffer heart disease. That's a huge price to pay.

We hear the whiny questions: Do I have to turn off the TV and go exercise? Can't I stay healthy without jogging? How important is exercise for me and my family? We could go on and on about physical fitness related to inactivity.

And just why do people not exercise? Many think we do not have time, that we have no or limited access to convenient facilities, that we do not feel safe in the environment where we could exercise. What is your excuse?

Schools and community organizations become ever more important in providing time, space, and safety for physical exercise. The Health Ahead/Heart Smart school health curriculum for elementary schools (Superkids/Superfit) emphasizes exercise along with general health and nutrition. For the youngest, lessons focus on the importance of stretching and warming up before vigorous activity, having fun through exercise, and performing physical activity to make hearts stronger and healthier. Progressively, youngsters learn other benefits – flexibility, muscular strength, and endurance, for example. They develop athletic skills and learn to create their own fitness activities. The concept of being active becomes an ingrained part of their routine; they know exercise is important to good health, and they know why and how it works.

Families still bear responsibility, too, for recognizing the need for active lifestyles and helping each other get off the couch and into the activity zone. Motivation toward movement – each can help the other.

Any parent who even tries to get the children up and moving can begin to claim role model status for his or her children. Physical activity can involve the whole family – walking, running, riding bicycles, swimming, or engaging in team sports such as softball or soccer. Take advantage of a natural ability for sports – yours and the child's; and remember that non-competitive exercises are fun, too!

The Centers for Disease Control and Prevention (CDC) advises adults who would be role models, especially people who have been inactive for awhile, to take a sensible approach by starting out slowly.

- Choose activities you enjoy, and you'll be more likely to stick with them. Gradually build up the time spent doing the activity by adding a few minutes every few days until you can comfortably perform a minimum recommended amount of activity (30 minutes per day). This isn't much of a problem for kids.
- As the minimum amount becomes easier, gradually increase either the length of time performing an activity or increase the intensity of the activity, or both.
- Vary your activities, both for interest and to broaden the range of benefits.
- Reward and acknowledge your efforts.
- Now, apply your gain as advice for children. That's what makes you a role model! For yourself, having a consistent companion or "trainer" might help, but exercise is what an individual must do to be healthy.

Planning physical activities for children requires understanding the unique nature of their bodies. Often adults whose expectations are too high are the ones responsible for organizing and supervising activities. Pressure, stress, and competition can cause otherwise enjoyable activities to become disastrous experiences that discourage continued physical activity. This is particularly a problem with competitive sports. Too vigorous, competitive sports can injure young, incompletely developed joints or muscles. Lack of success also hurts. Participate in Little League, but study the dynamics and stress by parents to win. Always consider non-competitive exercise, not just for athletes, among your options.

The pre-adolescent lacks complete development of fine motor control and hand-eye coordination. Appropriate athletic programs for this age include total body activities such as running, swimming, cycling, and hiking.

By pre-high school age, all of the body's long bones have not yet fused. Soccer, basketball, volleyball, and swimming are good sports for this age group.

High school students, especially those in their final two years, have almost entirely fused long bones; their bones are becoming fully calcified and growth is slower. That's when we can encourage competitive and contact sports, although many are not adequate for proper fitness. Standing around watching teammates play does not make a person fit. Look at some baseball players, for example. Some group activities in physical education do not promote fitness.

Again, adult pressure can *discourage* even the fun of simple running if the child is pushed beyond his or her limitations. And long-distance running can result in serious injuries. Early evidence shows that maturity and growth can be delayed in pre-pubertal children who engage in competitive long-distance running. Additionally, children might not be able to tolerate the high body temperature associated with distance running. Parents, coaches, and physicians should know such facts before allowing children to compete in ultra-strenuous activities. In hot weather, football practice can lead to dehydration and heatstroke; urge caution and be sure of adequate fluid intake and appropriate rest periods. Sadly, a doctor's son became overheated in early football practice. They put him in a hot shower, and he died of heat exhaustion. Cool down evenly with cold towels as needed. Beware of strenuous exercise in the hot summer.

Many adolescents lift weights to increase muscle mass. This isometric form of exercise can raise blood pressure to very high levels. Training with weight machines might achieve the same results without creating such blood pressure extremes. Occasionally, coaches encourage excessive weight gain and muscle-building to enhance the competitive edge; this can add to cardiovascular risk. Just look at the obesity in high school football players! Try to build muscle mass, not weight with fat.

What is fitness?

While different sports and exercise activities might develop one element of fitness over another, four elements comprise all-around fitness:

- cardio-respiratory endurance
- lean body composition
- flexibility
- strength

Cardio-respiratory endurance is the ability of a person's heart and lungs to exercise briskly for long periods of time without tiring and to be able to adjust to it without a great change in pulse rate. When fit, the heart muscle gets larger and beats more slowly but pumps a greater volume of blood with each contraction. At rest, the fit heart can deliver the same amount of oxygen with less work. During exercise, when the heart beats faster, it can deliver more oxygen to the muscles, thereby increasing endurance.

Someone with a fit cardio-respiratory system generally has about 10 percent more blood in his or her body but a relatively low blood pressure, partly because exercise opens the tiny blood vessels in the muscles and allows blood to flow more easily through them.

Exercise that requires a continuous supply of oxygen to the muscles – running, swimming, or dancing, for example – these are "aerobic." Dr. Kenneth Cooper, who coined the term, and his wife get credit for encouraging jogging. It has caught on. Aerobic activity can be sustained for hours, if the oxygen supply system – the heart, lungs and blood vessels – is up to the task. Thirty minutes to an hour a day is enough for fitness but might not be enough to reduce obesity.

People describe aerobic exercise as "huffing and puffing" exercise. Some argue as to how much huffing and puffing one needs before aerobic benefits begin to show. For a long time, the typical aerobic fitness prescription was to exercise at 70 to 80 percent of maximal heart rate (see below) for at least 20 minutes, three times a week. Now most experts believe prolonged endurance with more energy expenditure reduces heart disease and recommend exercise daily. In other words, an ideal fitness program consists of five-times-a-week sessions lasting 30 to 45 minutes each. Consistent exercise programs should start in elementary grades and really be encouraged in high school, when PE is often dropped.

Maximal heart rate varies from person to person and changes with age. A rough estimate can be figured by subtracting a person's current age from 220. The target pulse rate for a youngster of 10 would be 70 to 85 percent of 210 or about 150 to 180 beats a minute. This is just an approximation.

Another factor that comes into consideration is maximal aerobic power (which is sometimes called maximal aerobic capacity or maximal oxygen intake). These technical terms describe the point when the heart and circulatory system cannot deliver any more oxygen to the tissues, and one cannot exercise much longer or harder without approaching exhaustion. The usual recommendation is to exercise for a sustained period between 60 and 80 percent of maximal aerobic power. This is the "target zone." The two points – maximal aerobic power and maximal attainable heart rate – are very close.

The main point is to get up and start moving. Simply getting the heart rate higher than "resting" level outweighs worrying about whether a heart rate is at the level it should be. The body seems to know how hard the heart should beat.

Lean body composition reveals the percentage of a person's weight that is composed of lean body mass – muscles, bones and organs – compared to fat.

Flexibility refers to the ability to move each joint through its complete range of motion and to stretch muscles fully without causing damage. Flexibility gets a lot less attention than other aspects of fitness in children because people assume – incorrectly – that children are naturally flexible.

While youngsters are more flexible than adults, they are not tiny wind-up toys whose limbs easily rotate in 180-degree circles. Children should develop and maintain flexibility because they otherwise become pre-disposed to joint and muscle injuries in later life.

Proper stretching provides the key to maintaining flexibility. The bouncing and calisthenics you might recall from grade school days doesn't replace s-l-o-w stretching. Always stretch out muscles before beginning strenuous exercise and do stretches after.

Strength gives the muscles the ability to exert force against resistance. When a muscle is strong, each individual muscle cell is enlarged and contains more nutrients and a greater number of the tiny units that enable the muscle to contract. Contracting against resistance builds muscle strength. Isometric exercise builds strength and, importantly, bone structure. Bone structure in youth retards osteoporosis or bone thinning later in life.

A child must develop strength early to do simple things – standing up straight, for example. Muscle resistance exercises build different muscle groups as those in the arms and the legs, and that resistance complements aerobic activities.

Isometric exercises at a young age help prevent bone thinning and fractures later in life. This is particularly true for white females. Many exercises concentrate on legs and lower body, but the arms and upper body need isometric exercise, too. Both isometric and aerobic exercise are important to begin and continue from youth.

Having a ball, taking a walk

The American Heart Association declares physical inactivity to be "a major risk factor for cardiovascular disease, and most Americans are not physically active enough to gain any health benefit. Swimming, cycling, jogging, skiing, aerobic dancing, walking or many other activities can help your heart. Whether it's included in a structured exercise program or part of your daily routine, all physical activity adds up to a healthier heart."

A couple of children in Mississippi, reportedly the fattest state in the nation, developed their own "Just Have a Ball" project. During their first three months, according to a local TV news report, they garnered and gave more than 4,000 balls to other children. These kick balls, basketballs, soccer balls, and footballs got kids moving, resulting in more exercise, less pent-up stress and, probably, weight loss or helping to maintain ideal weight.

Having fun and being physically active result in physical and emotional benefits. Increased physical activity can reduce the risk for many diseases – including cardiovascular disease, some cancers, arthritis, type 2 diabetes, and depression. Being physically active also can help with losing or maintaining weight, strengthening bones and muscles, and preventing falls.

With a little creativity and planning, even adults with the busiest schedule can make room for physical activity. For many people, the most ideal time to cycle, walk, or play is after meals, school, or work. Think about a weekly or daily schedule and look for or make opportunities to be more active. Try to pick a consistent time. Even keeping a log book can help. A log or notes on cards is a great incentive.

Every little bit helps. Consider the following suggestions from CDC:

- Walk, cycle, jog, or skate to work, school, the store, or place of worship.
- Park the car farther away from your destination.
- Get on or off the bus several blocks away.
- Take the stairs instead of the elevator or escalator.
- Play with children or pets.
- Take fitness breaks – walking or doing desk exercises – instead of taking cigarette or coffee breaks.

- Perform gardening or home repair activities.
- Avoid some labor-saving devices – turn off the self-propel option on your lawn mower or vacuum cleaner.
- Use leg power – take small trips on foot to get your body moving.
- Exercise while watching TV (for example, use hand weights, stationary bicycle/treadmill/stair climber or stretch).
- Take family walks, but remember: each person exercises to his own capacity.
- Dance to music.
- Keep a pair of comfortable walking or running shoes in your car and office, and you'll be ready for activity wherever you go!
- Make a Saturday morning walk a group habit.
- Walk to do errands.

As an aside, always remember to keep safety first. For example, don't permit children to go on walks alone after dark or take the stairs in a poorly lit building. There are always other ways to achieve fitness goals.

For adults, set aside just 30 minutes to start, and every day get out and move; mix some isometrics with aerobics. Set the example!

Chapter Nine

How to cope, like yourself, manage stress

When the going gets rough, adults often long to return to the simple pleasures of childhood. But is the age of innocence *really* a time of simple pleasures? Or do children face just as wide a range of stressful situations as adults?

A new mother, Lucy holds up her beautiful seven-month-old and teases, "It's not easy being a baby, is it?" She's right on target. While that particular baby lacks for nothing, most infants and toddlers worldwide suffer untold traumas and tragedies during their childhood.

Many children, for example, must cope with parental divorce and all the fears and uncertainties of having a single parent. Divorce might also mean parents develop new relationships, possible marriages, and step-relations. Change can also mean moving away from a familiar home, going to a new school and church, saying good-bye to the familiar, and having to build new friendships.

Even within the so-called nuclear family, a child must deal with many pressures: the physical and psychological changes of growing up, possible dangerous people in the neighborhood, unsafe situations at school, and persistent problems caused by sex, drugs, and alcohol.

Another major source of stress for many children is the pressure to "do well." Parents, teachers, and coaches, as well as peers, exert so many performance expectations: win all the games, dress fashionably, be popular. Achieve, achieve, achieve!

Competition's long been the *practice* in most American schools, starting from kindergarten. And competing with other children goes beyond getting the gold stars; children are encouraged to compete with themselves to be the best they possibly can. For some children, adopting this attitude at a very early age can lead to a spiral in which they seldom – if ever – feel satisfied with their achievements. This stress often contributes to illness and disease!

A child's stress is not your stress

Trying to judge stress in children has been difficult without precise tools to evaluate anxiety. Most often, the best method is simply to ask the child how he or she feels toward a specific event or activity. Take time to talk it out. You as the adult can then observe the child's possible stress-related behaviors. Sometimes talking together can relieve stress.

A child clinical psychologist studied nearly 700 children aged 12 to 14 and concluded that children and adults have very different perceptions of what constitutes a stressful event and how stressful a given situation is. Jeanne E. Dise-Lewis, PhD, developed an inventory of more than a hundred potentially stressful life events for children, arranging them in order of stressfulness. These ten stressors top the list:

- One of your parents died.
- A close family member died.
- Your parents decided to get a divorce.
- Your mom or dad was put into jail.
- You were picked up by the police.
- You were suspended from school.
- Your mom or dad moved out of your home.
- You got caught stealing something.
- You had to move in with relatives or into a foster home.
- A friend or someone else close to you died.

Does any of these apply to your child? If not, that's good. But how about "your family had financial problems," ranked 16th, or "your parents had a fight or argument with each other," which is ranked at 64. Or "all your homework got piled up at once along with other work," number 25, or "your parent embarrassed you," which ranks 58th.

Yes – stress exists everywhere for children. Stress lurks in the classroom, in the family kitchen, on the way home from school or shopping, even in the mirror. Growing up is hard to do!

A body versus stress

Both children and adults react physically to stress. When the body senses an acute threat – real or perceived – it prepares itself to either fight or flee. Medically speaking, these are the things that happen when a body is under stress:

- The cerebral cortex in the brain sends a message through our nerve networks to alert the body to prepare for the stressor.
- The heart beats faster, and blood begins to circulate more efficiently to provide additional fuel for a quick reaction.
- Skeletal muscles, especially those required for quick motion, tense in preparation for confrontation with the stressor.
- Additional oxygen is routed to the brain to stimulate thought processes.
- Eyesight and sense of smell are sharpened in response to impulses sent from the cerebral cortex.
- The adrenal glands contract, sending out adrenaline and causing skin to redden, especially in the facial area, and blood sugar levels to rise, resulting in quick energy burst.
- Airways leading to the lungs open wide for the deep breathing necessary in vigorous physical activity.
- Blood with red blood cells is pumped faster, providing oxygen to the muscles in the limbs.
- Chemicals are released in the skeletal muscles to reduce fatigue and allow for sustained, long-term rigorous activity.

- Chemicals enter the blood stream to accelerate blood clotting in case of injury.
- Nerve impulses signal the bladder and bowels to empty, which is why some people wet their pants during extreme fear.

What does stress look like?

Nobody can see nerve impulses, glands contracting, or airways dilating. So how do you know when your body is responding to stress? What are the most telling indications that the fight-or-flight response is turned on?

Many signals exist: rapid pulse, increased perspiration, pounding heart, tightened stomach, shortness of breath, gritting teeth or clenching jaw, racing thoughts, an inability to stay still.

Most of the time, these reactions are short-lived. They only prepare the body to lash out at an attacker or run away from a dangerous situation. When the stress-provoking situation is removed or resolved, the body returns to normal.

Sometimes, though, the situation is not one of physical danger but rather of anger or frustration. As an adult, for example, you miss out on a job you want. You might have no socially-acceptable way to release the pent-up fight or flee reactions; so your body experiences a tremendous amount of wear and tear. If such situations occur routinely, the body stays in a state of chronic stress. In return, chronic stress can cause illness.

You might wonder why this topic is included in a book about improving childhood health and providing answers to how you can "fix the fat." According to a study at Cedars Mount Sinai Medical Center in Los Angeles, mental stress can directly affect the heart. In one task, researchers asked participants to perform rapid mental arithmetic. In another, they had to give a speech about their own flaws. And when speaking about their faults, people showed heart abnormalities almost as pronounced as those produced by vigorous physical exercise, such as riding a stationary bicycle to the point of exhaustion.

Think about that when your child gets nervous about his or her math test. Do not just give the off-handed answer, "Oh, you'll do fine." While we aim for this book to help your child develop the self-esteem that allows him or her to stop thinking of certain personality traits or inabilities as "bad," you as a parent must remember that everyone sometimes needs a good "ear." Do whatever you can to keep yourself and your children "at ease" – that's the opposite of *dis*-ease!

Your child might not tell you about his or her pounding heart or knot-in-the-stomach. How can you know the kid's troubled or anxious? Some signals are the lack of enthusiasm for everything; inability to play or have fun; sleeping problems, bed wetting, listlessness, complaints about feeling tired or bored; inability to concentrate; poor appetite, weight loss; crying, sulkiness, irritability; constant fidgeting; whining about un-verifiable physical ailments; and – worst of all – references to death and suicide.

While these signals are usually an alert to chronic stress, they might also mask depression, a very serious problem, especially in adolescence. Dr. Hans Selye from Montreal coined the word stress over 60 years ago but said we are always under stress. It is how we handle stress, and that is called *dis*-tress.

No more Type-A

Everyone experiences stress – from the moment of birth. But some people deal with stress very differently than others.

During the 1970s, a theory emerged that had to do with the so-called "Type A Personality." A complex set of behaviors characterize Type A coronary-prone behavior: extreme aggressiveness, competitiveness, easily aroused hostility and impatience. In some adult studies, Type A behavior has been associated with coronary heart disease. Type A behavior was considered a product of environmental influences: parents, teachers, and cultural factors. Early identification of this kind of behavior could lead to the development of programs to modify this behavior. Over the next decade, questions arose over the validity and usefulness of the theory.

Today we know that people who talk fast and always hurry are no more likely to die from stress than people who are laid-back and soft-spoken. Those who are hostile and angry, however, can claim increased risk for stress-related disease. Being hostile is a villain.

Lawyers, doctors, and community-active people – all have come under the watchful eye of internationally acclaimed experts in behavioral medicine. The research from Duke University Medical School by Redford Williams, MD, and Virginia Williams, PhD, revealed that such factors as paranoia – *"People are picking on me;"* social avoidance – *"I'd rather not meet that person;"* and even workaholism – *"I love working 15 hours a day"* do not correlate with early death. Findings also showed that personality traits that reflect cynical mistrust – *"People lie to get ahead,"* anger – *"I'd like to kill that person,"* and acting from anger – *"I'll just give that person a few punches (or stabs or bullets) to make him understand"* – do strongly predict premature death of heart attack.

Famous philosopher and comedian Will Rogers claimed to not dislike anyone he ever met. Gosh! I wish I were like that, but – *sorry* – I am not. I am human, and anger and inward feelings are part of me.

Cynicism and anger emerge in hundreds of everyday situations. Standing in a checkout line that moves too slowly – because some people have more than the allotted number of items – can generate feelings of anger as well as actual angry confrontations. Over time, people get into the habit of feeling angry over factors that are beyond their control – such as the weather, traffic tie-ups, their lack of money, the high cost of gas and groceries – that they *live* in an unpleasant state. That might drastically shorten their lifespan!

Angry, hostile behavior begins in the early years. When we factored our children studies on Type A and B behavior (our Hunter-Wolf scale), hostility related adversely with risk factors. Children in late elementary school can exhibit symptoms noticeable to the observant parent or teacher. The responsible adult will take action to help the child modify thoughts and actions toward behavior change and, possibly, extended life expectancy. Encouragement and local rewards can go a long way. We know anxiety and distress are harmful, and relaxation exercises are very helpful.

Several activities described in the Health Ahead/Heart Smart program can help deal with stress. One such lesson plan suggests the individual describe "floating on a cloud."

Another way is to teach kids to develop friends – with good social habits, of course. You and your children need others with whom you can "talk it out." If you cannot embrace friends willing to share feelings, then maybe you need a psychiatrist, and that's both expensive and not always as helpful as a sympathetic ear. Make the time to spend quality time with your children and other family. Listen to what they say and answer their questions with honesty, sincerity, and respect. Know, too, that as you age, you will find your friends die off, and you have no one to talk to. Don't let loneliness affect you or your children; don't let stress become distress.

Chapter Ten
Arnold's story: *learn from him*

The boy from Bogalusa who grew up to become "Doctor Gerald Heart Smart" always loved to find answers that could solve real-life problems. Now a grandfather, Doctor Gerald entertains his young grandchildren with captivating stories and the lessons learned from his experiences. One such story is as follows:

I was sitting in my office one day and in walked a woman looking very anxious.

"Are you Doctor Heart Smart?" she asked.

In my medical practice – unlike in research and teaching – I'm known in the community as Dr. Heart Smart (*at least for this book*).

"It's my overweight husband Arnold. He's near death with diabetes in your hospital. Please, can you tell me how to help get him well? I just don't know where to turn,'" she cried. "He is so young – just a few years out of college. This happened so suddenly, so unexpectedly. I can't rest until I can begin to understand. Then, maybe then, we can get him back on his feet and in good health again."

I listened to her story.

"My name is Andrea," she began. "I met Arnold four years ago and we got married just six weeks after meeting. Poor Arnold – he never did know how to say 'no' to an éclair or a raspberry tart. His fingers are stained from holding cigarettes, and he never exercises, always watching

TV and football games. Anyway, when I came home yesterday, there he was, slumped over in his chair, a bag of potato chips on the table beside him and a milkshake in his hand."

I promised Andrea I would do what I could to find out more about Arnold's illness, but I had my suspicions. I assigned names to the likely suspects:

- ✓ **Opal Obesity**
- ✓ **Lite Larry**
- ✓ **Harry Heart Disease**
- ✓ **Arthur Atherosclerosis**
- ✓ **Howard Hypertension**

This is what I explained to Andrea:

"Opal Obesity might not look as though she could do much harm, but she's killed countless people with heart disease, diabetes, and other illnesses. The worst thing about Opal is that she sneaks up on you. As a matter of fact, more than a third of the people in the United States are in Opal's clutches right now – *they're fat!* And not even in the category they call "obesity."

"Opal is not hard to find, either. She likes to hang out everywhere people consume too many calories and get too little exercise. One of her favorite weapons is fat in food because fat contains, ounce for ounce, more than twice as many calories as carbohydrates or protein. She also likes sugar – candy, cakes, cookies, pies, and soft drinks. All have corn starch and high fructose sugar.

"Anyone who wants to avoid severe illness, such as Arnold's, must avoid those high-calorie and empty calorie concoctions – the treats with oily, slick, slippery sugary toppings. Instead, stick with foods that are typically low in calories, like fresh fruits and vegetables or foods that have been modified to be low in calories. We don't even know if all the sugar substitutes are safe being consumed from childhood.

"Some folks think it's safe to hang out with **Lite Larry**, but Lite can mean just about anything. No standard exists for that word, but we do have standards for 'low cal' or 'reduced calorie.' Lite can refer to the amount of salt, as in corn chips, or the color of a product, such as lite chocolate, or to the amount of corn syrup, as in lite fruit cocktails. So just because the word 'lite' happens to appear, you cannot be sure that the product will be lower in calories."

Andrea and I took a break and walked over to a local snack shop. There on the menu, large as life, was granola. Many people think of granola as a health food. *Beware!* We tout it for fiber, but look at the calories. Just plain old fruits and vegetables help that along with grains. Watch out when we see refined.

I continued my instruction on healthy food.

"Believe it or not, Andrea, granola is high in grams of fat and high in sugar. A single bowl has three tablespoons of fat and three tablespoons of sugar. When Opal learned the federal government lists her sugar weapon as an ingredient on food labels, she began to use aliases – different names where she can hide without being detected. That's one of the tricks of marketing. But you can find her hiding under such names as sucrose, fructose, dextrose, corn syrup, honey, maltose, molasses, apple juice sweeteners, maple sugar, sorbitol, and brown sugar. And while sugars – by whatever name – add on pounds, they also sit on your teeth, waiting to be attacked by bacteria. In diabetes, excess sugar in the blood (increased hemoglobin A/C) affects small blood vessels; that causes eye and kidney problems. Blindness, starting with eye troubles and silent kidney disease, is a companion of diabetes.

"But Opal didn't work alone on Arnold. **Harry Heart Disease** and **Arthur Atherosclerosis** helped her. Harry and Arthur have two favorite weapons: saturated fat and cholesterol. Saturated fat can raise the portion of your blood cholesterol, called low-density lipoprotein cholesterol (LDL-C) that deposits killer clumps of plaque in your arteries. The more plaque, clots occur; and the smaller the opening and the harder for blood to get through. Finally, blood that carries oxygen to the heart, and without which the heart cannot live, can no longer get through. Many times these plaques rupture and produce a clot that closes off the vessel causing what we call 'sudden death.'

"The problem with saturated fat is that it's hard to track because it's hidden in many foods. But I do have good news. The federal government has located Harry and Arthur and has identified them in many of the foods you buy in the supermarket. They're listed right there on the label: coconut oil, palm oil, cocoa oil, hydrogenated oil, lard, butter, shortening, whole milk, cream, and vegetable shortening. *They all mean fat!* It's in candy bars, granola, yogurt-covered raisins, popcorn, and chips. *Gosh! Do I like a bag of popcorn in the picture show?!* And remember, fat was big in that bag of chips you found next to your husband.

"You also have to consider cholesterol, though it's not always listed by that name on the label. You can tell, though, because cholesterol exists *only* in foods that come from an animal – foods such as fat meat, eggs, cheese, and whole milk. We are learning how to limit this and, especially, the saturated fat."

Yet another suspect remained on my list: **Howard Hypertension**. Howie has been known to work alongside Opal Obesity, Lite Larry, Harry Heart Disease, and Arthur Atherosclerosis on big jobs known as heart attacks. Sometimes, he'll work alone on jobs called strokes.

"Howie's biggest weapon is sodium. He's got a ton of aliases: salt, MSG, brine, broth, baking soda, soy sauce, and baking powder. If you find any of these aliases among the first five listings on a product label, better watch out. Canned products almost always mean high salt. Excess salt (sodium) is a real danger. Howard has his eye on you – he's right there in that TV dinner, the Chinese take-out meal, the pickle, the soups and the canned vegetables. Salt and obesity are the big weapons that cause hypertension. (*Earlier we discussed micronutrients of sodium, potassium, magnesium, and calcium. Trace amounts of zinc, copper, and selenium are important, and the need for iron can easily be judged by blood studies*)."

So, there were the possible culprits, my list of most likely suspects who might have gotten Arnold in trouble. *But which one contributed most?*

To learn more, I visited my colleague in the hospital laboratory. He showed me charts, x-rays, and slides that were taken of Arnold's arteries. We decided that Arnold has had too many rounds of junk food. An interesting aside is that we now know that central and upper body fat and obesity have a strong relation to diabetes, coronary heart disease, and high blood pressure. Liken the human body to pieces of fruit: the pear and feminine body configuration, and the apple or the upper body male configuration, such as his bulge over his beltline. A healthy waist measurement should be below 40 inches for adult men and 35 inches for women. Even those are liberal measurements! Men tend to have heart disease 10 years earlier than women. Getting down to a lower weight and a body mass index of less than 25 is critically important. Proper, adequate nutrition and exercise – walking, swimming, sit-ups – can help him achieve that goal.

"But hopefully that's not the end of the story. To help him get healthy, get the family involved. Everybody in the family can help the others find and reduce Opal Obesity, Lite Larry, Harry Heart Disease, Arthur Atherosclerosis, and Howard Hypertension. Many have the same problem as poor, sick Arnold. Take someone grocery shopping with you to make sure that your basket does not fill up with cakes, candies, pies, soft drinks, fatty foods and salt!

"And while you're watching out for the bad foods, you can also look for healthy helpers – fiber, protein, and the complex carbohydrates or unrefined grains. Always look for the serving size and how many servings you'll get out of the package, how many calories are in a serving, and how much protein and carbohydrate. Fiber is also important, particularly soluble fiber. Unfortunately, labeling is often lacking the information on soluble fiber."

I went back to Andrea and told her what I had found out about Arnold. I told her that she should use her new knowledge about food so that she can stay healthy and get her husband back on the road to good health. Now she will look to beans, lentils, barley, whole unrefined rice, sweet potatoes, leafy vegetables, fruit, and even some nuts, as her friends.

Andrea promised that she and Arnold will start a joint exercise program. They'll walk every day, enjoy the pool in warm weather, do their own yard work, and plant a small vegetable garden. She also said she wants Arnold to quit smoking and for both of them to quit or dramatically cut back on drinking alcoholic beverages. Even light beer and wine calories can soar out of control!

All those changes will be a challenge, and probably neither Andrea nor Arnold will be able to make food changes, exercise, stop smoking, and reduce drinking all at once. But if they are determined to change their lifestyle, they will become healthier over time.

"Also, Andrea, think about what effect all of this will have on your children."

They start out as little Arnolds.

Chapter Eleven
Pitfalls can hamper good intent, behavior

"Behave!"

What mother or dad, grandparent, older sibling, or other-adult-in-charge has not at least at one time in her or his experience stared directly into the face of a child and hissed, "Behave!"?

The scolding remains consistent: be nice, act appropriately, consider others, take care of yourself and beware of potential predators. Humans "behave" when they manage their actions in a particular way, when they conduct themselves properly.

Parents who aim to grow "Heart Smart" babies – and infants and toddlers in families just like yours – more likely will verbalize that admonition for generations to come. Their own families have learned how they can grow heart-healthy children from the cradle well into adulthood. Those youngsters – and others with determination to prevent heart disease – can *choose to behave* for healthy days ahead. You, too, must behave differently to fix the fat – to adjust, change, diminish, lose, repair – so that you can achieve best health, including getting obesity firmly under control.

What does your family's behavior reveal about you?

Do you get enough sleep, or do you fall asleep at your desk or the wheel of your car? Do you eat nutritious food and appropriate portions? Do you abstain from tobacco and all tobacco-related products? Do you walk, run, cycle, or play ball, or do you lump yourself like a potato on the couch? TV is so appealing – as are computer games, movies, and other non-participatory events!

Do you get "upset" easily and frequently?

Can a good balance of activity and leisure exist?

Certainly!

Children and adults alike should aim for at least 30 minutes of vigorous exercise every day and also set aside some quiet time for meditation, reading, or just listening. Individuals should think about and choose daily behaviors that will benefit them.

Following such a "balanced" lifestyle – much more, embarking on a brand new set of rules to live by – might be very difficult for some. Awareness of the pitfalls that you can confront can go a long way toward resolving fears and strengthening discipline.

- **Pitfall number one**: People will not necessarily change their behavior even if they believe their lives are threatened. If they would, cigarette sales would have hit zero long ago. To give up smoking habits 20 to 30 years in the making remains a very difficult task. For children never to start smoking would yield a much better outcome. Stop the experimenter and encourage early quitting.

- **Pitfall number two**: Reducing a single risk factor is not as effective as reducing multiple risk factors. All risk factors link together as if each were tied to or tangled with all the others. Such tight interaction results in their nasty tendency to gang up on an individual! Blood pressure tends to increase as weight goes up, and as weight goes up, cholesterol levels might rise, too. People who seldom exercise often are overweight and also have high levels of a "bad" cholesterol. Exercise helps to raise good cholesterol. This prompts many physicians to talk about "lifestyle" changes instead of centering on any single risk factor.

Based on your and your child's risk factor profile, you might need more exercise and to modify your diet. The more good habits, the longer and healthier life you can anticipate. A 45-year-old man who has adopted three changes could increase expected lifespan to about age 78; not too long ago, that was age 67 – *quite a difference!* For women, an average of 82 years has been reached. Fortunately, whatever we are doing, thanks to education by the American Heart Association and National Institutes of Health, our lifespans have gradually increased.

But – and this is a *BIG* but – how many men or women do you know who will adopt six or seven of these good changes? If someone is exercising two or three times a week, for example, he or she probably does so at the expense of an extra hour or two of sleep a night or skimping on breakfast on exercise days. Even worse, one might schedule seven hours' sleep a night – most people would have no problem with that – but at the expense of the exercise . . . and often breakfast, too. Is this the model we want for our children?

- **Pitfall number three**: Reducing risk factors will protect an individual against heart disease but not affect a total cure. Some of this is not new. We continue to cite older studies, though, because the findings have survived the test of time.

Occasionally, research findings irritate some in the scientific community. While some agree that lowering cholesterol could save lives, for example, they emphasize that the one factor will not cure heart disease. Furthermore, one study proved only that drugs could effectively lower cholesterol – *not* that adopting a new, healthier diet late in life would do so. Even if that were possible, they argued, getting the American public to forego fried eggs and bacon, stacks of pancakes, buttered, and lots of good maple syrup, fatty hamburgers and French fries, and fatty ribeye steaks likely would not happen. But you can adjust with moderation.

Adults *can* be successful in changing lifestyles and approach a risk-free status. But starting in adulthood cannot achieve maximum prevention – much better to begin as a child! Start teaching kids healthy decision-making.

Young children develop attitudes and behaviors within the family setting. As they extend their environment beyond the family, behaviors change in response to peer pressure, increasing awareness, and various life influences. Adopting healthy lifestyles leads to good health behavior later and affects health, longevity, and quality of life. At a young age, children can be inoculated against adopting unhealthy lifestyles such as cigarette smoking and illicit drug use while they also learn what constitutes a good general lifestyle.

Conclusion

The best result for your having read – and continuing to use – this book as your and your family's encouragement to heart health is that you have dedicated yourself to making the present and future lives of your children healthier, safer, and more fulfilling. A healthy child is a better student and, later in life, a more positive member of society – a better citizen, a happier individual.

Young children begin to develop attitudes and behaviors at birth, from the crib onward. Please, therefore, teach your children from the earliest that adopting healthy lifestyle choices, healthy decision-making, and learning to take responsibility for their own bodies is not just a choice but a *necessity*.

The health of your children – *our children* – is our country's present and future!

Appendix
About Health Ahead/Heart Smart

Knowledge gained in the Bogalusa Heart Study has been applied to develop, test, and evaluate methods for cardiovascular risk and to begin prevention. Investigators of the Tulane Center for Cardiovascular Health, the Tulane University Health Science Center, the Louisiana State University School of Medicine, University of New Orleans, and the Jefferson and Orleans Parish School Systems collaborated to develop a comprehensive program for elementary school children Called "Health Ahead/Heart Smart." This represents a broad, coordinated health education and promotion program that is a result of the first NIH-appointed National Research and Demonstration Center – Arteriosclerosis.

The Health Ahead/Heart Smart (HA/HS) school health curriculum, already in use in many schools helps develop methods needed for children to adopt healthy lifestyles. The curriculum encourages children to learn health concepts, develop healthy attitudes, and adopt the necessary skills and behaviors that will ultimately reduce their cardiovascular risk, obesity, and diabetes. This model needs to be adopted by parents and growing children who face the environment in which they will grow.

Health Ahead/Heart Smart – Program of Health Education for Elementary School Age Children (K-6) – can be accessed on the Internet (see http://www.som.tulane.edu/cardiohealth/ahead.html) for parents to also use with children in the home. Even you as parents and role models can benefit because the material is intended to help you and teachers extend health promotion lessons into the community.

Lesson plans follow an educational calendar of growth as children get older and move into higher grades. A proper "scope and sequence" (or growth in education plans) is very important for development of the teaching concepts, both within grades and across grade levels, as shown in the following table:

Scope and Sequence

	General Health	Nutrition	Exercise	Psychosocial	"It's Me"
K	Locate and name body parts. Explore five senses.	Recognize healthy vegetables, fruits, "Food Stores" game, variety of food tastings; Field Trip Yogurt Parlor.	Importance of stretching and warming up the body for activity. Develop an awareness of how group games can enhance physical fitness through fun and excitement. Perform a physical activity to make hearts stronger and healthier; identify benefits of exercise.	Demonstrate personal hygiene regarding hand-washing, mouth care, bathing, and sleeping.	Recognize similarities and differences, phone number, and address. Learn respect, "words to live by." Earn self-esteem.
1	Identify size, location, and role of the heart; examine emotional and physical changes since birth; function of skeleton and muscles; determine health enhancing behavior.	Role of food, taste-test new foods; function of nutrients in the body.	Benefits of feeling fit and promoting self-esteem internal and external fitness; fitness for everyone.	Recognize and differentiate emotions; recognize ability to change feelings.	Learning to share and work with others; recognize differences in family structure; identifying trusted adults; identify situations when students feel afraid.

2	Importance of rules at home and school; problem which face other with handicapping condition; positive aspects of medicine, trusted adults; resisting peer pressure.	Making healthy choices; recognize variety; peer support for healthy choices; awareness of problems of hunger and homelessness.	Caring for others is a part of heart health; develop personal fitness through patriotic songs and movements.	Reinforce identification of emotions and connection between external emotions; influence of events on behavior and feelings.	Explore variety of feelings, skills to select and maintain friends; recognition for special events and successes.
3	Identify communicable and non-communicable diseases; personal responsibility for health, and the world in which we live; apply concepts learned to make healthy choices.	Protecting the balance of the eco-system; preserving food sources; recognizing healthy foods; pledge to promote personal health.	Fitness for everyone, through dance and locomotive movement; promotion of flexibility, muscular strength, and endurance.	Develop inter-dependence on thought and positive self-esteem; identify appropriate and inappropriate criticism.	All people make a difference; reinforce skills of collaboration selecting different methods for reacting to difficult situations; alternatives to fighting.

4	Identify location of the heart anatomy and physiology of the cardiovascular system; identify major risk factors of heart disease, high blood pressure, high blood cholesterol, smoking, and contributing factors of stress and lack of exercise; identify characteristics of health-enhancing behaviors; physiologic or smoking.	Demonstrate ability to follow a recipe; identify food high in fat, salt, sugar, identify four basic food groups; plan healthy meal and snacks; prepare CV healthy foods; classify foods in four food groups.	Understand the role of exercise in heart; demonstrate the three stages of a workout (warm-up, bout, and cool-down); identify the components of physical fitness; understand frequency, duration and time; develop an awareness of how group games can enhance physical fitness through fun and enjoyment; understand the benefits of exercise on daily life; develop and monitor an individual fitness program; understand the effect of different exercises and activities on heart rate.	Characteristics of good health; identify power, personal strength; D.E.C.I.D.E. Model; combating inappropriate response patterns; self-reinforcement, improved self-esteem; identifying stress, overcoming stress.	Identify characteristics of enthusiasm; importance of positive attitude, impact of peers and role models on behavior, examine importance of names and labels; use positive imagery to create a feeling of success; identify steps in achieving goals.

5	Identify specialized function of veins and arteries; smoking effects; concepts of wellness; reinforce anatomy and physiology of cardiovascular system.	Distinguish between saturated and unsaturated fats; log and measure food quantities; analyze food labels; classify foods; determine physiological effects of sugar, fat, and salt on CV system; monitor food intake.	Describe relationship of cardiovascular disease and physical fitness; define components of physical fitness; design, monitor, and maintain an individual fitness program; demonstrate correct form and technique for various fitness activities (jogging, aerobic dance movements, jump rope, etc.); develop a mind set toward exercise; identify additional benefits of aerobic exercise; calculate and monitor heart rate to express intensity of individual workout; develop personal decision-making skills related to fitness activities.	Reinforce previous concepts; identify "triggers," cues, and consequences; define empowerment; identify motivational strategies for self improvement; resisting peer pressure; improving coping strategies.	Identify how attitude affects performance, identify personal successes, create feelings of empowerment; identify verbal and non-verbal cues; examine responsibilities.

6				
Reinforce above concepts; experiment measuring blood pressures, identify various types of heart disease components of blood, red blood cells, white blood cells, plasma, and platelets, unalterable risk factors (heredity, sex, race, and age).	Adjust caloric intake as needed; select healthy items in a restaurant; model heart-healthy food selection for peers; examine the importance of complex carbohydrate. Choose CV-healthy foods when dining out; energy expenditure and balance.	Reinforce exercise concepts; introduce exercise physiology (oxygen utilization, specifically of training); identify major muscle groups, prime movers associated with specific exercise; free choice jogging distance; soft impact aerobic dance; care and prevention of fitness-related injuries; perform individual aerobic activities; stretch-walking; internal training; reciprocal aerobics, cardiovascular contract workout.	Maintenance of concepts learned; identify positive role models; demonstrate sending accurate messages; solicit peer support; identify passive, assertive behavior; act assertively with peers.	Influence of roles models, characteristics that make individuals unique; evaluation of judgments, apply visualization techniques, effective communication skills. Develop social responsibility. Analyze goal setting and visualization techniques.

Children begin in the early grades to learn rudimentary ideas, such as location of body parts and that the heart is a pump, and about blood cells. Such exposure provides the beginning of understanding and dispelling of fear of one's own body. Concepts of good nutrition and need for physical activity are begun and emphasized. Compassion and relationships are begun. The concepts develop as the child progresses through the elementary grades. By 6th grade the youngster, for example, has a good working knowledge of cardiovascular anatomy and physiology. The kids understand what blood pressure is, and each can practice taking blood pressure with a sphygmomanometer on themselves and on their parents. Results might not be accurate, but the attention focuses on hypertension and beginning prevention and learning good social behavior.

Such development of knowledge and understanding accompanying the child's growth and development is an important educational tool — and a unique aspect of the HA/HS curriculum. The curriculum is age or grade-specific to address cognitive processes appropriate to each child's age.

To ensure continuity among grades, the curriculum includes transitional material in all module areas. For example, in the area of nutrition, transitional material serves to shift the emphasis in earlier grades of identifying "healthy" foods to a more sophisticated understanding of the physiologic effects of sugar, fat, and sodium.

Further, in each grade the curriculum begins with an introductory review lesson that allows implementation in all grades as a new school begins the health education program. Importantly, consideration is given for introducing the curriculum into new schools at all grades. The more personnel involved in grades K-6, the more powerful the intervention can be. Older students provide role models for younger students, and all develop a knowledge base of cardiovascular and general health. Reviews provide a bridge of learning between old and new knowledge.

Materials' format

Readers can encourage their schools to consider incorporating the HA/HS curriculum, which includes a self-explanatory "Teacher's Guide" with rationale, introduction to a health curriculum and grade focus, and lesson plans. Each lesson plan includes the focus, background information if needed, objectives, key words, materials needed, suggested dialogue and resource material, additional illustrations and accompanying materials, and student worksheets. The best way to approach prevention is through health education for children. Yet a family can begin to understand the depth and scope of information related to achieving a healthy growth through using such lesson plans.

❖ *Integration into the academic agenda* — The HA/HS curriculum is appropriate for teaching in the social living, health, or science time period and in physical education classes. The "It's Me" module can be taught in social studies classes to students who are receiving the complete curriculum. This allows for a broader involvement of teachers and emphasizes social learning. Within a given elementary school, students may be "departmentalized," which implies that a single teacher covers certain subjects to all children in a particular grade rather than all subjects to just one group of students.

❖ *Delivery of curriculum* — Although all teachers preferably would teach the curriculum, when only one teacher is selected to teach the curriculum, other teachers are encouraged to participate. They can do so by teaching the "It's Me" module, using the supplementary "Teacher's Guide," involving their classes in physical activity (Superkids/Superfit with many non-competitive activities), helping with afternoon "perk-ups" and geographic fun runs, taking part in the school lunch intervention, and enrolling in after-school teacher aerobic dance classes, which also provide behavioral skills — shopping for food, dining out, cooking, and smoking clinics, for example. These are just part of the activities.

❖ *Time required* — The curriculum was developed for 25 to 30 contact hours per school year, with lessons being taught approximately 30 minutes three times weekly. Obviously, this will be modified by teachers, depending upon their acceptance of the importance of teaching aspects of health and how the lesson plans can be interpreted into other subject areas.

The strength of the HA/HS curriculum is that, while directed to heart disease, it also recognizes the other problems facing education today. Using social cognitive principles, self-efficacy, and teaching self-esteem beginning in kindergarten introduces the inoculation concept against unhealthy lifestyles.

In this manner, changes in the school environment — for example, an improved and more nutritious school lunch and the addition of more, non-competitive physical education for individuals — are supported and, in turn, the environmental changes bolster teaching concepts in the curriculum. The empowerment concept encourages children to feel confident in their abilities, to choose between positive and negative alternatives, sing songs about being healthy, and achieve mastery experiences while receiving support from teachers, parents, and peers. All reinforce the adoption of healthy lifestyles.

Summary of concepts: learning healthy behaviors

The national focus on early childhood education must begin with the health of every child. This includes being well-nourished, activity-oriented, and prepared to learn. The key to developing such children starts in the home and involves the whole community in which children can grow and thrive.

Researchers from the BHS have been studying, writing, and publishing scientific information about cardiovascular diseases since 1975. No fewer than 1,000 scholarly articles have been published in addition to contributions to some 50 book chapters and the publication of five books!

Beyond, the team of BHS professionals continues to practice what they teach and preach. The senior author — nearing his ninth decade of life — continues 150-mile round-trip weekly treks to Bogalusa for the Study and works tirelessly from his office in Tulane University's School of Public Health and Tropical Medicine and also tries to exercise daily.

So, does this Health Ahead/Heart Smart method offer families the proverbial "magic bullet?"

No!

No trick can guarantee a successful health promotion program. The only answer is that an individual, a family, must decide and dedicate the effort to make the present and future healthier, safer, and more fulfilling. A successful effort must involve the child, parents, medical and education communities, and other family and friends.

Over the years with funding from whatever source became available, the BHS developed, produced, and implemented excellent teaching materials for elementary schools. By the mid-1980s, the HA/HS K-6 Health Ahead/Heart Smart Curriculum emerged from the BHS. Based on a "medical school-university-community preventive education model, HA/HS became a joint project of the Tulane Center for Cardiovascular Health, Tulane and LSU Medical Centers, Jefferson Parish, and New Orleans School Systems and the Louisiana Office of Public Health. Schools participating in the curriculum pilot encouraged parent participation; involved students in school-wide activities; sponsored a school-based health fair; and conducted physical activity and nutrition assessments. Lessons were integrated into math, science, social studies, art, and music.

HA/HS relies on scientific data on how people adopt and employ new ideas and behaviors in their own lives. It is made to be teacher friendly. Each lesson contains lesson goal(s), measurable objectives, suggested support materials, suggested student assessment, lesson background information, suggested teacher dialogue, student activities, and in-home activities for students to share with their family members. In-class and in-home activity sheets and parent letters are provided for convenient reproduction.

HA/HS relies on theoretical constructs from research in how people adopt and employ new ideas and behaviors in their own lives. Readers who want to fully explore this further might study the PRECEDE Model (Green, et al., 1980) and Albert Bandura's Social Cognitive Theory for motivation concepts. Bandura believed that "human functioning is the product of a dynamic interplay of personal, behavioral, and environmental influences," and the HA/HS health education program relies on that concept to achieve desired results.

Simplified so parents can put the program to use in their daily lives at home, the program considers three kinds of factors that affect "fitness" in youngsters:

❖ Predisposing — Individuals can choose which knowledge, attitudes, beliefs, perceptions, and values they embrace and practice.

❖ Enabling — Individuals can decide to get a health screening and then use the resources and learn the skills necessary to strengthen "good" behaviors and change "bad" risk factors.

❖ Reinforcing — Individuals can achieve rewards for performance toward avoiding risk factors and achieving good behaviors.

Bandura said his theory is this: *"People plan courses of action, anticipate their likely consequences, and set goals and challenges for themselves to motivate, guide and regulate their activities. After adopting personal standards, people regulate their own motivation and behavior by the positive and negative consequences they produce for themselves. They do things that give them satisfaction and a sense of self-worth, and refrain from actions that evoke self-devaluative reactions. The human capacity for self-management is an aspect of the theory that makes it particularly apt to the changing times. The accelerated pace of informational, social and technological changes has placed a premium on people's capabilities to exert a strong hand in their own self-renewal and functioning through the life course."*

In addition to good nutrition and an emphasis on fitness, the HA/HS curriculum emphasizes self-esteem, being positive about oneself. Beginning in kindergarten, or even at the pre-school age, children are encouraged to have respect for their bodies and to respect teachers, parents, and other professionals. Having a good attitude and learning to make wise decisions become ever more important! Hands-on activities and learning healthy choices are part of the curriculum.

Equally importantly, the curriculum addresses such social problems as drugs, alcohol abuse, sexually transmitted diseases, dropping out of school, and violent behavior, even bullying. The program aims to give children's health and behavior (lifestyles) a boost that will last them a lifetime! HA/HS strongly advocates that a healthy child is a more effective student and, later in life, a more positive member of society.

The parish, the governmental entity also known as a county, in which Bogalusa is located adopted the curriculum to improve health for all children parish-wide. Washington Parish (County) aims to assess the health problems of children (approximately 7,000 elementary school children) and develop programs that can improve the health of children in a parish-wide area as a model for other parishes in Louisiana as well as in other states. In one school in Franklinton, Louisiana, Regina Delatte kept records of sixth through eighth grade students. Some lost weight. The weight gain expected for growth of children at this age over a semester is 5 pounds. The school average was 1.7 pounds. In using the President Futures Challenge, a quarter mile run started at 3.5 minutes and decreased to 2.5 minutes for the average.

Medical, public health, education, and citizen residents of this parish are encouraged to address several problem areas: control and prevention of obesity; improved asthma-bronchitis treatment and follow-up; completed vaccination programs; dealing with drug and alcohol abuse and tobacco use; and to address such social issues as sexually transmitted diseases, teenage pregnancies, violent behavior, and suicides.

This background statement convinced Washington Parish that something needed to be done in their schools:

> *The BHS has documented medical and social issues that involve the health of children. Many of these are preventable, and they have a detrimental effect not only on the health of growing children but also on the economy of the community. Improving health of children and individuals throughout the Parish can be accomplished by planning and implementing already available programs.*
>
> *Although the Bogalusa Heart Study focused primarily on cardiovascular diseases, it became obvious that children and young*

adults followed over the past 30 years have developed preventable medical problems, not only heart disease but other medical, dental, and social problems. These disabilities can be prevented by helping young individuals achieve healthy lifestyles, not only through nutrition and physical activity but also by understanding the damaging effect of unhealthy lifestyles such as use of excessive alcohol, tobacco use, inactivity, and poor diets leading to obesity and increasing diabetes.

Importantly, the program begins in kindergarten. However, too few schools use such a curriculum nationwide, and too few teachers and parents know how to teach and reinforce health education. If you do not have direct access through your school to the HA/HS program, you can obtain the program and adjust it for home use (see resource at the end of this book).

Another intervention model involved families with known risk factors. This instructional design involves implementation conducted by a multi-disciplinary team of a cardiologist, psychologist or counselor, nutritionist, an exercise specialist, and a nurse specialist to help organize the program. Even with the abundance of information from other sources, professionals from the BHS Group offer its science-based education curriculum for physical activity and exercise for teachers and children.

More about Health Ahead/Heart Smart

When is the latest time you sat with your child, expressed your love, and said how good he or she is? That precious time is important to you both! One-on-one interaction proves to the child that "me" matters.

"Healthy self-esteem is a child's armor against the challenges of the world," asserts the home page of KidsHealth, the self-proclaimed "largest and most-visited site on the Web providing doctor-approved health information about children from before birth through adolescence." Created by The Nemours Foundation's Center for Children's Health Media, the award-winning site provides families with accurate, up-to-date, and jargon-free health information they can use.

Schools and children using the HA/HS curriculum focus on the self-esteem armor from kindergarten through grade six. For example, the curriculum for the youngest includes five lessons:

- ❖ *I Am Special* — Discussing how each student is unique, but also similar to other students.
- ❖ *More I Am Special* — Promoting the importance of knowing one's own address and phone number.
- ❖ *Your Name is Special* — Encouraging students to recognize and write their own names.
- ❖ *Don't Talk to Strangers* — Discussing who strangers are and when to go to trusted adults.
- ❖ *Growing Like Me* — Discussing how kids' bodies grow just like plants and animals and how to promote healthy growth.

Through instruction, interaction, practice, and talking with family at home, youngsters build self-confidence. They feel good about themselves. They can be happy and optimistic because they know they can handle the situation or know how to ask for help.

As they grow and the lessons intensify, the foundation of "feel good about me" builds to influence attitude, motivation, behavior, and strong emotional adjustment.

Both educators and family participate with growing children. All can contribute to the positive growth and development in different ways. Adults must see themselves as role models and remember that small children often have big ears. Your words and actions, what you say and what you do, the reasons you give for the choices you yourself make — all influence youngsters.

While children do listen and watch, they also want to be heard and seen. **Make the time to spend quality time with your children. Listen to what they say and answer their questions with honesty, sincerity, and respect.** No, the nine-year-old is not yet an adult. But that child's way of thinking and feeling responds to how he or she thinks you as an adult feel about and behave toward him or her. While you might sometimes need to correct your child, do so with care and encouragement that such a mess-up or mistake probably will not happen again.

Create a relationship and a home environment that both protects and nurtures the child. Let the child know in words and actions that your home has "heart," and that the heart is safe and healthy.

If you have trouble or doubt about parenting skills, ask for help. You might need a mentor — somebody older, or even younger, than yourself who has "been there, done that." Seek assistance, guidance, and patience to give your child the best you can. Grandparents can play a role, too, in addition to just "baby sitting."

Communicate your needs; change to improve however you can; but don't sweat what you cannot change. Be the best parent you can.

Just participation makes a winner. Not everyone can be the outstanding starter, but the little ones help create a beautiful home environment and a healthy future!

From another direction, we also include "words to live by." These include compassion, respect, love, kindness, consideration — each supported in the HA/HS curriculum.

Choosing a healthy lifestyle — in many, if not most, cases — actually costs less in time and money than taking the "fast-food," "couch potato," unplanned way of life. Prevention almost always costs less than cure. New estimates show that with early prevention people can actually save money by reducing doctor and hospital visits and taking fewer medications.

The HA/HS curriculum is divided into five sections: General Health, Nutrition, Exercise, Psychosocial, and It's Me. Each lesson can stand alone or be incorporated to complement the existing grade level health education program. Initial curriculum evaluation documented that teaching a majority of the lessons from each section achieved the greatest health benefits. Therefore, teachers are encouraged to teach as many lessons from each of the five sections as possible.

- **General Health:** To stress that health is a personal responsibility to be worked on each day by making healthy choices and practicing healthy behaviors.

- **Nutrition:** To learn the importance of eating healthy foods at home, at school, and when eating out. Using the Department of Agriculture's Food Guide Pyramid or food plate, students assess their typical eating patterns and that of their family's. Students also learn about foods from other cultures around the world.

- **Exercise:** To become more aware of the relationship among regular physical activity and personal health/wellness. Students participate in non-competitive games and practice warm-up and cool-down with each physical activity. Schools are encouraged to participate in the program "All Children Exercising Simultaneously Around the World" (ACES).

- **Psychosocial:** To understand the importance of effective communication in resolving conflict and to develop coping skills. Students role-play strategies to promote positive peer influence through assertive behavior in response to intimidation and aggression and practice stress reduction and ways to avoid violent behavior. They learn to adopt healthy lifestyles by coping with pressure, including resisting smoking, alcohol and drug use, and staying in school.

- **It's Me:** To become aware of his/her own special skill(s) and talent(s) which make him/her unique. By emphasizing self-esteem, students are encouraged to celebrate and share their special skills and talents and to appreciate and respect the uniqueness of others. In respecting themselves, students are better able to refuse behaviors that endanger optimal wellness and encourage healthy attitudes and values.

The HA/HS program is a comprehensive initiative that addresses the entire school environment — lifestyle changes for teachers, changes in the cafeteria, and increasing physical activity for all children, not just athletes. The program includes 75 non-competitive exercises and a physical education curriculum.

The message that this program conveys is simple: *eat sensibly, be physically active, practice healthy behaviors, and achieve good attitudes and human values.* The curriculum's impact is measured by the ability of students to practice health protective behaviors while taking responsibility for their own health. This is called *empowerment.* Importantly, HA/HS addresses all components of the school environment with teacher's guides for the classroom, a manual for improving nutrition, exercise concepts of fun, non-competitive physical education for all children, and programs involving parents and teachers as role models.

Addressing physical activity

Superkids/Superfit is an integral part of HA/HS. Developed by physical education specialists (primarily by Steve Virgilio, PhD, at the University of New Orleans, now at Adelphi University in New York, and his graduate students), this component encourages *all* children to participate and enjoy *non-competitive* physical activity, regardless of athletic abilities. These activities stress the importance of maintaining regular physical activity throughout one's lifetime. The program encourages physical activity for all children, not just athletes, as a lifelong routine for fun. Competitive and team sports are good since they use activities and teach cooperation and social behavior, but these are not for all kids.

Superkids/Superfit is "user friendly." School systems using the comprehensive health education curriculum know about its easy-to-use Guidebook and Activity Box, with oodles of non-competitive activities for school children. Any teacher regardless of physical training will find Superkids/Superfit worthwhile. Since the program requires minimum equipment and space, teachers can apply it to any environment: walk, jog, ride a bicycle, and swim, for example.

While competitive sports like soccer, basketball, and football are great for aerobic activity, as with all sports, injuries become part of the game. That's why teachers or assistants at school and adults at community- or home-based activities must pay attention to the youngsters and the exercises they choose. Teaching children "safe play habits" and the need to drink plenty of water while working out are good lessons for their lifetimes. Also to be considered is being careful with excessive activity during days with high temperature.

The BHS Group developed the "Superkids/Superfit" physical education program to encourage lifelong physical activity for fun. In the United States, children seem to be adopting a sedentary lifestyle at earlier ages. Observations from the BHS show children watch two to six hours of TV every day. Now add the time spent at the computer and playing electronic games. Not nearly enough children participate in physical activities — time that historically occurred among children themselves or through such community organizations as YMCAs, churches or synagogues, or private health clubs. The average child actually spends more time watching TV than being in the classroom, even though child health experts recommend no more than one to two hours of TV a day for youngsters over age two — for the younger ones, no "screen time," according to some experts.

Adult pressure can discourage even the fun of simple running if the child is pushed beyond his or her limitations. Early evidence shows that maturity and growth can be delayed in pre-pubertal children who engage in competitive long-distance running. Additionally, children might not be able to tolerate the high body temperature associated with distance running. Parents, coaches, and physicians should know such facts before allowing children to compete in ultra strenuous activities.

Keeping exercise an enjoyable activity to be done on a regular basis should prompt all to vary the routine and to also remember that the development of non-competitive, personally achievable goals often provides the kind of self-reinforcement many people need to remain motivated.

With a few keystrokes — "exercise" — and a mouse click on "enter," Google delivers some 202 million Internet sources for exercise. Not every site provides what you might enjoy or need, *certainly not all at once!* But many highly regarded government agencies, not-for-profit associations, health related businesses, and publishers offer something for everyone. Much of this is for adults, but adults set the example for children.

The *It's Me* curriculum

Ricky Laahty, a famous carver of the Zuni Pueblo in southern New Mexico, draws acclaim for his special productions, "frogs with an attitude." Most of the little animal figures are believed to have magical powers to protect or aid their owners. Their whimsical expressions always bring smiles to fans. Collectors consider a "frog with an attitude" to be a good thing.

But not all people experience a smiley-faced attitude. Some, in fact, with high risk factors for serious diseases live with negative or even hostile states of mind. Additionally, they lack the self-esteem needed to embark on a healthy lifestyle course.

Beyond general health, nutrition, and exercise components, the HA/ HS Program offers two additional tracks: psychosocial and *"It's Me."* Lessons integrate national health education, science, and technology standards and follow physical activity, nutrition, and tobacco use prevention guidelines recommended by the CDC. We believe the psychosocial and self-esteem lessons often get lost in the rush of daily life. That's unfortunate. A major aspect of the program is teaching children self-esteem; teaching them to feel good about themselves; and to begin taking care of their health early in life.

The *"It's Me"* section within the HS/HA curriculum contains lessons and activities that are designed to enable students to develop self-knowledge, social responsibility, personal power, and an enhanced self-esteem. This teaching begins in kindergarten.

The component intentionally tries to help students take a new look at the different ways that ideas are received. Too often, individuals unconditionally accept the "norms." The *"It's Me"* curriculum aims to help students in the "inoculation" process against learned helplessness. This "inoculation" is similar to the process in which a doctor would provide a vaccination against a disease or to assist the biological processes.

"It's Me" provides the same type of defense for students by helping them become aware of the forces that affect their lives; to act responsibly to themselves and others as well as the environment.

Now, turn that around for your own children, and make *"It's Me"* a family affair starting in kindergarten and even earlier. The program encourages empowerment and healthy attitudes — respect for others, respect for their own bodies, respect for teachers and parents and peers. Starting health education early can motivate children to be better students and community residents. By emphasizing self-esteem and knowledge about healthy lifestyles and behavioral skills, an education program can become basic to the prevention of disease in adulthood.

The program encourages young children to develop proper decision-making skills and the opportunity to learn coping skills that will prevent the adoption of unhealthy lifestyles. A good educational program can counteract bad influences — such as those learned at home, from peers, or via mass media that encourage adoption of unhealthy lifestyles — and even help reverse them. A set of healthy "words to live by" are provided — respect, lovingly, honor, integrity, etc.

Within the psychosocial module are lessons that teach assertiveness, problem-solving, and coping skills such as inoculation against peer pressure that encourages smoking, substance abuse, and other negative health and personal behaviors. For example, the "DECIDE" module uses a decision-making strategy that is taught and the children practice in role-play situations. This is taken from Lawrence Green, a noted health educator. The DECIDE model acronym, cited in an article in *The Health Care Manager Journal*, comes from six particular activities children need in the decision-making process:

D = define the problem

E = establish the criteria

C = consider all the alternatives

I = identify the best alternative

D = develop and implement a plan of action, and

E = evaluate and monitor the solution and feedback when necessary.

Additionally, in this part of the curriculum, students learn the physiologic effects of smoking and how to identify advertising ploys. They practice assertive behavior involved in refusing cigarettes. Such role rehearsal coupled with social support of classmates helps empower students to transfer the classroom practice to real-life situations. Play acting and TV taping for playback is a good tool. An example to record is having a child refuse cigarette smoking encouraged by a classmate.

Children need to learn the importance of coping with stress and practice relaxation skills. One lesson plan asks the student to describe floating on a cloud. Encourage and practice identifying physiologic stress sensations, and through progressive muscle relaxation, visualization, and imagery techniques, learn ways to cope with environmental stressors. An important aspect of the behavior skills taught in the educational component is the use of empowerment techniques. Children need to be encouraged to consider personal positive qualities and features. Children record positive attributes and recall previous and current accomplishments to enhance confidence in their abilities. It's all about "little steps for little people." When teachers can reinforce these concepts in interactions with students, or parents with their children, then it becomes a powerful tool to motivate and encourage children for learning and adherence to the goals of healthy behaviors.

Another program encourages parents and the community to be involved with newsletters and health fairs. For example, there are geographic fun runs across the country with a big United States map that shows the progress of each participant. Along the way, runners can talk about the historical sites they "pass," as well as the cultural features of special area, such as the Alamo or Carlsbad Caverns. Mathematics also can be integrated, and "racers" can learn to take heart and pulse rates. The thrust of the program is behavioral orientation, starting in kindergarten.

Readers who would like the program considered for their elementary school can see that the comprehensive health education program addresses general health of the entire school environment. The newly revised edition of the curriculum integrates national health education, science, and technology standards and also incorporates school guidelines for nutrition, physical activity, and tobacco prevention recommended by the CDC. Lessons have been revised to include measurable objectives, valid assessments, technology resources, additional student activities, and in-home application activities.

What this means to you

These "lessons learned" and you-can-do-it-too guidance come from a comprehensive health promotion program based on the BHS and can show you and your family how to choose and achieve heart health.

From this book, we encourage you to develop sensible rules and give clear instructions — learn to communicate, particularly with youngsters. Learn how to avoid bad behavior before it happens, to practice and demonstrate good, heart-healthy behaviors.

Go to it! We encourage you to do so. Just do it.

About the authors

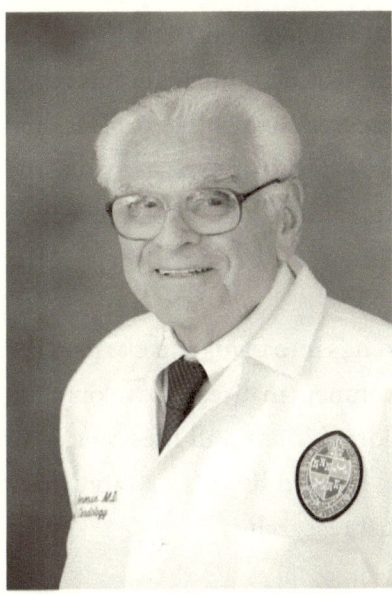

Gerald S. Berenson, MD

A native of Bogalusa, Louisiana, Gerald S. Berenson is a graduate of Tulane University and the Tulane School of Medicine. He has taught as a cardiologist at both Louisiana State University and Tulane University Medical Schools for over 40 years. He was section chief of Cardiology at LSU Medical Center for 17 years.

His primary interest is in atherosclerosis, coronary artery disease, and hypertension, and he is the principal investigator of the Bogalusa Heart Study, which has become known nationally and internationally for the study of the early natural history of heart disease. As an outgrowth of their observations of poor lifestyles, unhealthy diet, smoking, and inactivity contributing to obesity, he and his colleagues developed a prevention program for elementary school children, the Health Ahead/Heart Smart health education program, and a Family Health Program to control cardiovascular risk factors. Dr. Berenson's interest is in the prevention of heart disease, and he encourages health education of children and families as a public health approach for preventive cardiology. He and his group have published more than 1,000 journal articles and five books documenting his research.

Gerald Berenson was the initial recipient in 1997 of the Council for Young Children's Kids First Award of New Orleans. Tulane honored him with its Outstanding Alumnus Award in 1999 and a Tulane 50th anniversary Lifetime Achievement Award in 1995. In 2005 he received the Meritorious Achievement Award of the American Heart Association (AHA) for his contributions to understanding the early origins of atherosclerosis in childhood; and in 2006 he was the recipient of the AHA's Population Research Prize. In 2008 he received a Distinguished Scientist award of AHA. A widely sought visiting scholar, lecturer, and conference leader, Dr. Berenson has ably served many other professional organizations, including the American Society of Hypertension, the American College of Cardiology, and American Society for Preventive Cardiology; he is a Fellow of the American Association for the Advancement of Science.

Berenson brought some disturbing trends into focus and clarified the complex interactions of genetics and environment in disease development. The national emphasis on healthier children's diets and lifestyles is, to a large extent, predicated on the lessons learned by this extraordinary clinician-scientist from a lifetime of robust research.

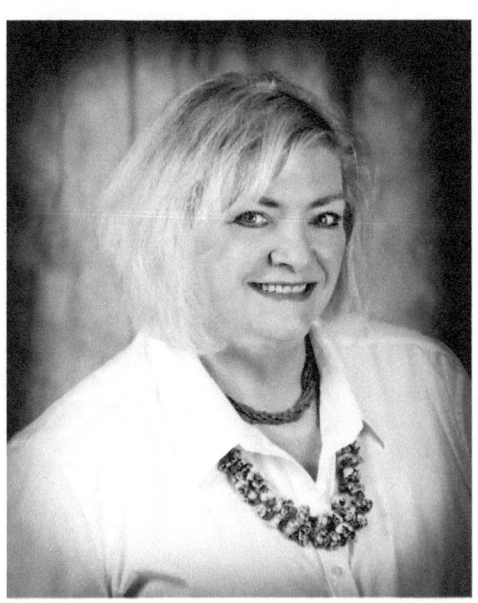

NancyKay Sullivan Wessman continues her communications career as a solo practitioner, offering public relations consultation and services through Wess*Comm*, LLC, and as a freelance writer and editor.

A newspaper journalist early, she worked nearly 25 years as director of communications and public relations for Mississippi's statewide public health agency. She is a founding member of the National Public Health Information Coalition,

NancyKay Sullivan Wessman, MPH

a graduate of Tulane University School of Public Health and Tropical Medicine with a master's degree in public health, a charter member of the Tulane SPHTM Alumni Association Board of Directors, and a communications consultant to several federal agencies and national organizations.

The Mississippi native lives in Jackson and intermittently writes two blogs. As Mizrizbaboo, at www.mizrizbaboo.wordpress.com, she writes about her personal "renew, reinvent, revolutionize kick [that] has to do with mind, body, computer, kitchen, personal and public personages, and whatever else flits through my mind during a given post." Wessman Words, www.WessmanWords.com, marks her "movement toward a new career, change to a writer's life, shift to centering on word power. Current projects reside firmly in the nonfiction realm, and both books-in-process revolve around public health."

Glossary

Angina pectoris – angina means pain; pectoris, in chest area; associated with coronary artery disease

Ischemia – inadequate blood supply to heart

Atherosclerosis – "hardening" of the arteries, disease of lining of arteries, leading to heart attack, peripheral artery disease, and occlusion in other arteries

Fatty streak, fibrous plaques – lesions occurring as part of atherosclerosis

Blood pressure (systolic, top figure; diastolic, bottom figure) – pressure in arteries

Hypertension – high blood pressure, disease producing damage to target organs (organs served by blood vessels), for example, heart, kidney, eye, brain

Body Mass Index (BMI) – weight/height^2, measure used to evaluate overweight and obesity

Clustering – aggregation, grouping, and interrelationship of risk factors

Diabetes mellitus – metabolic derangement involving insulin, glucose, and various hormones; often with hypertension; abnormal lipids; damages large and small blood vessels

Insulin — hormone produced in pancreas controlling blood sugar level and utilization by muscles and cells

Insulin resistance — often with obesity

Epidemic – large population involvement with disease

Family tree – characteristics of individual family members and how related

Height – expressed in inches, meters, or centimeters

Incidence – frequency of developing disease

Lipids, lipoproteins

- **Total cholesterol** — cholesterol is a yellow dry powder; total cholesterol exists in various substances like lipoproteins to be made soluble

- **Lipoproteins** — mixture of proteins, cholesterol, phosphorus, solubilizes cholesterol so it can be carried in blood

- **Low density lipoprotein cholesterol (LDL-C)** — has highest amount of cholesterol ("bad" cholesterol); this is deposited in vessels to form atherosclerosis

- **High density lipoprotein cholesterol (HDL-C)** — "good" cholesterol triglycerides – fatty acids and some cholesterol, rises after fatty meal in blood, occurs mostly in very low density lipoprotein cholesterol (VLDL-C)

Metabolic syndrome — mixture or cluster of four risk factors – central body (abdomen) fatness, insulin resistance, hypertension, hyper-triglycerides, now more complex as cardiometabolic syndrome

Myocardial infarction — heart attack, coronary vessel occluded

Overweight, obesity – excessive body weight

Percentile — Percentage of a risk factor or variable in the population – example, 10th percentile or 50th percentile, etc; 95th percentile often used to be abnormal

Risk factor – characteristic or variable producing risk of heart disease – examples, hypertension, high cholesterol, or diabetes

Saturated fat – fatty acids with no double bond $(CH_2 - CH_2 - CH_2 - ...)$

Unsaturated fat – fatty acids with double bonds $(CH_2 - CH_2 = CH_2 - ...)$, can not be produced by the body; occur as mono or poly

Tracking – Persistence of a risk factor over time – remaining in a rank relative to the population levels

Weight – weight of body, measured in pounds (lbs) or kilograms (grams)

Resources

American Heart Association –
www.americanheart.org

Berenson, Gerald S. *Causation of Cardiovascular Risk Factors in Children: Perspectives on Cardiovascular Risk in Early Life.* New York: Raven, 1986. Print.

Berenson, Gerald S. *Evolution of Cardio-metabolic Risk from Birth to Middle Age: The Bogalusa Heart Study.* Dordrecht: Springer, 2011. Print.

Berenson, Gerald S. *Introduction of Comprehensive Health Promotion for Elementary Schools: The Health Ahead/Heart Smart Program.* New York: Vantage, 1998. Print.

Centers for Disease Control and Prevention –
www.cdc.gov/growthcharts
www.cdc.gov/HealthyYouth/tobacco/facts.htm
www.cdc.gov/nccdphp/dnpa/healthyweight/assessing/bmi/index
www.cdc.gov/nccdphp/dnpa/nutrition/nutrition_for_everyone/basics.
www.cdc.gov/nccdphp/dnpa/physical/everyone/index
www.cdc.gov/nccdphp/dnpa/physical/everyone/get_active/index.htm

Choose To Move –
www.choosetomove.org

"Couch-potato Culture May Cut Our Lives Short." *MSNBC.com.* Web.
www.sys12-nbcsports.msnbc.com/id/23358982/page/2

Doctor Gourmet –
www.drgourmet.com

Framingham Heart Study –
www.framinghamheartstudy.org/risk/index.htm

Georgia State University –
www.gsu.edu/~wwwche

Healthy People 2020 –
www.healthypeople.gov/2020/about/DefaultPressRelease.pdf
www.healthypeople.gov/Document/HTML/Volume2/19Nutrition.
htm
www.healthypeople.gov/2010/LHI
www.healthypeople.gov/2020/default.aspx
www.healthypeople.gov/2020/LHI/nutrition.aspx

McMahan CA, Gidding SS, Malcom GT, Tracy RE, Strong JP, McGill HC
Jr; Pathobiological Determinants of Atherosclerosis in Youth Research
Group. Pathobiological determinants of atherosclerosis in youth risk
scores are associated with early and advanced atherosclerosis. Pediatrics.
2006;118:1447-1455. Abstract

Medscape –
www.medscape.com/viewarticle/726173_print
www.medscape.com/viewarticle/758312_print

National Heart, Lung, & Blood Institute – National Institutes of Health
www.nhlbi.nih.gov/about/framingham/riskabs.htm
www.nhlbi.nih.gov/guidelines/obesity/bmi_tbl.pdf
www.nhlbi.nih.gov/guidelines/obesity/

National Library of Medicine –
www.nlm.nih.gov/medlineplus/cholesterol.html

President's Council on Physical Fitness and Sports –
www.fitness.gov/resources/facts/index.html

The Weight of The Nation –
http://theweightofthenation.hbo.com/films/trailer

Tulane University –
www.tulane.edu/som/cardiohealth
www.tulane.edu/som/cardiovascular/index.cfm
www.som.tulane.edu/cardiohealth/default.html
www.som.tulane.edu/cardiohealth/supkid.html

"Women & Heart Disease Fact Sheet." *WomenHeart:*. Web. www.
womenheart.org/resources/cvdfactsheet.cfm

www.ingramcontent.com/pod-product-compliance
Lightning Source LLC
Chambersburg PA
CBHW020439290526
45785CB00002B/931